I0091532

Catharine with an A

Edna Keir

Catharine with an *A*

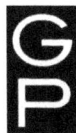

GP

To the memory of Noel

Catharine with an A
ISBN 978 1 74027 222 3
Copyright © Edna Keir 2003

First published 2003
Reprinted 2016

GINNINDERRA PRESS
PO Box 3461 Port Adelaide 5015
www.ginninderrapress.com.au

Contents

Foreword

This is a testimony of what true love and dedication has accomplished for Catharine, our Down syndrome daughter. She is now aged thirty-six. I have written her story to place on record the considerable role that the family, primarily her brothers and sister, have played in Catharine's development and in her many achievements throughout her life.

My hope is that others may be assisted and encouraged by our experiences.

I sincerely wish to thank Joan Dwyer of the Fellowship of Australian Writers, Lambing Flat Regional, and all who assisted me in this venture.

A Special Child

A meeting was held quite far from earth.
It's time again for another birth.
Said the angels to the Lord above,
'This special child will need much love.
Her progress may seem very slow,
Accomplishments, she may not show,
And she'll require extra care
From the folks she meets down there.
She may not run or laugh or play,
Her thoughts may seem quite far away,
In many ways, she won't adapt,
And she'll be known as handicapped.
Oh, let's be careful where she's sent,
We want this life to be content.
Please, Lord, find parents who
Will do a special job for you.
They will not realise right away
The leading role they have to play.
But with the child sent from above
Comes stronger faith and richer love.
And soon they'll know the privilege given
In caring for this gift from Heaven.
Their precious charge, so meek and mild,
Is Heaven's very special child.'

Lisa from Victoria

1
The Birth

'We are praying that your baby is taken straight to heaven – it would be for the best.'

The values I learned during my early life, I believe, enabled me to cope with the emotional shock of hearing these words spoken to me in my late thirties.

From an early age, I had learned the importance of family values, a sense of humour, a strong faith, learning to live within one's means and the power of prayer. During my teens, I prayed that I would know and have the courage to follow my true vocation in life. Later, when the Second World War ended and I had met and fallen in love with a handsome young man just out of the air force, my prayer was that, if marriage was the vocation for me, I would become a good wife and mother (I have since added grandmother), that we be blessed with children and have a long, happy life together.

Fifty years later, I am thanking God, as he has answered my prayer in his own time and way. That young air force man was Noel Keir. He became a loving, supportive husband and father. We were blessed with six children, all of whom we are justly proud of, and now have seventeen grandchildren.

We were married with a Nuptial Mass in St Laurence's Catholic Church, Forbes, on 28th May 1949. With little money, but absolute trust in God and each other, we set out with joy and confidence on the journey of life together. We settled at 'Frankfield', a property near Bribbaree on the south-west slopes of New South Wales.

In the second year of our marriage, we were blessed with our first son, Michael, and two years later John was born. My next pregnancy ended with miscarriage. Then came Maryann, our first daughter. Michael had turned five and John was three. My mother was one of twelve children, Dad one of six, and I one of six. So, to me, three was only a start. Within the following four years, we had two more boys, Peter and Vincent.

Soon all but the youngest were at school; the two eldest boys at boarding school. As a mother, I felt incomplete without a babe in arms and a toddler underfoot. The children too began to ask, 'When are we getting another baby?'

On one of our rare trips to town – quite an occasion, taken mainly when Noel or I needed a haircut, or to visit a doctor or dentist – we met a friend with a new baby in a pram. As we chatted and admired the infant, Peter (aged six) could not keep his eyes or hands off the child.

'Don't touch her, Peter – she might wake up and cry!' said the new mother as she gently moved his hands away.

On returning home, after tea and baths were done, I took Peter aside to talk about the incident, as I knew his feelings had been hurt. 'It isn't nice to handle tiny babies,' I explained. 'Your hands might not be clean and could make a baby sick.'

'Well!' he said grumpily. 'If you would get one, I wouldn't have to be gawking at other people's, would I?'

I was certainly taken aback and, giving him a hug, I said, 'We'll have to ask God about that, won't we!' and tucked him into bed.

After some time, at age thirty-seven, I did become pregnant. Noel and I were delighted and wanted to spread the news, but agreed that Michael and John should be the first to know. The end-of-year speech night and concert at their college was only weeks away. We would be attending, and bringing the boys home afterwards, so we decided to wait and tell them in person instead of by letter.

On the homeward journey, with the three youngest asleep in the back of our station wagon, I broached the subject. 'Boys, Dad and I have something to tell you,' I began.

'You're going to have a baby, I suppose?' came from the back seat.

I was speechless for an instant. 'How did you know?'

'Just guessed,' came the reply.

'Well, what do you think about it?'

'It's all right, I s'pose,' was the non-committal answer.

We wondered how two big boys would feel about having a pregnant mum, but they just took it in their stride.

At about my eighth week, there was a German measles epidemic at the local school, and our children came out in spots. As I wasn't sure if I had ever been infected, I rang my doctor for advice. He decided to inoculate me, saying, 'This is just to be on the safe side!' This practice has since been discontinued.

My pregnancy continued normally, and anticipation mounted as my size increased. It was a very happy family experience, with so much love and attention showered on me by them all. I had always felt special when pregnant, but this time more so.

One day Peter, the ever-affectionate young lad, put his arms around my expanding tummy.

'What are you up to?' I teased.

'Just giving my baby a cuddle,' he said, quite seriously.

Three weeks before the expected delivery date, John was home for school holidays. We drove into Young to visit Michael, who was a patient in the Mercy Hospital, being treated for a duodenal ulcer. As I alighted from the car, I caught my heel in the hem of my skirt and tumbled onto my knees. There was no obvious damage apart from torn stockings and grazed knees. Early the following morning, I was disturbed from sleep with mild contractions. My earlier deliveries had all been induced when I was two and three weeks overdue, so this was quite unexpected – perhaps it was from the fall.

We had intended to go to Mass at Bribbaree that morning, 19th May 1966, as it was Ascension Thursday. Because we lived so far from town and were not sure how quickly things might evolve, Noel lost little time in getting the children organised and leaving John to milk the cows and generally take charge while he drove me to the hospital. Before leaving town, Noel picked up a television set on six months' rental, which would help to keep

11

the children occupied whilst I was away. This was their first experience of having television at home.

The day dragged on slowly, with no further progress. I wished we hadn't acted so hastily. 'Perhaps this was a false alarm!' I mused. After all, I was not due for another three weeks at least. But no, by 9 p.m. I went into full labour, and baby was delivered at about 10 that night.

I will always remember hearing the doctor saying, 'You have a little girl!' What a thrill – deep down, I had secretly hoped for a girl, but knew from experience that it would not matter. It seemed to take a little time for the doctor to get her breathing. I heard him instruct the nurse to prepare the humidicrib, but then say, 'Don't worry, nurse. She's OK – she wouldn't fit in it, in any case.' Moments later, she was shown to me for a short time.

'Those kids will love you,' I said, touching her chubby cheek. As it transpired, truer words have never been spoken. In my tired, blissful state, I did not notice any irregularity in her appearance and, on being returned to the ward I shared with another new mother, I drifted off to sleep after murmuring, 'A little girl. Thank you, God.'

However, the events of the next few days are etched in my mind.

My room-mate greeted me early in the morning. 'Good morning! Well, what did you have?'

'A girl,' I answered happily. 'My family will be delighted. I can't wait to see them. I wonder, do they know yet?'

As I tucked into breakfast, I kept imagining the excitement that must be erupting at home. Maryann would be thrilled to have a sister.

We went through the usual morning routine in preparation for feed time. I had done this all before, so knew just what to expect. My room-mate's baby was a few days old, so she joined the mums on the veranda in the sun. I waited patiently for my baby to be brought to me.

In those days, the babies were cared for in the nursery by staff members only, and they were brought into the wards for feeding. This was accepted as being necessary to protect our babies from infections that might be about during those fragile first days. But as time passed with no sign of anyone,

I supposed that they were busy, and baby was sleeping. I contented myself without a care – all was well with my world.

Eventually, Reverend Mother, whom I knew well, appeared in the doorway.

'Good morning, Sister,' I greeted her cheerily.

'Good morning, dear,' was her reply, with a tense smile on her face, and no congratulations. She *must* know our baby girl had arrived, and how pleased we would be? 'What time are you expecting Noel and the children, dear?' she enquired.

'I'm not sure, Sister. Some time before lunch, I expect,' I replied, puzzled by her approach.

Then came the bombshell! 'Doctor needs to talk to Noel, as there is a problem with the baby. I cannot say any more, but Doctor will tell you when he comes.'

I looked at her dumbfounded.

She continued. 'We are praying that your baby be taken straight to Heaven. It would be for the best!' She patted my hand and left with tears in her eyes.

I sat in stunned silence, lost in confused thought. Whatever could Sister mean? Our baby is fine. Didn't I see her myself last night? Or did I dream that! I am sure I saw her. She had a fat little face and a mop of dark hair. She was just fine. Sister was mistaken; she had the wrong person.

A little later, a priest came to me and said, 'Good morning, Mrs Keir. I am Father Bateman.'

'Good morning, Father,' I greeted him.

'We would like to baptise your baby – she isn't strong. We don't expect anything to happen to her immediately, but it would be best to baptise her just in case,' the priest explained in his quiet, gentle manner.

It must be true, I thought.

'Have you chosen a name for her?' he asked.

'Yes, Father. Catharine Bridget.'

'That is a good name!' he said. 'Is there anyone you would like to have stand with her that we could get this morning?'

My mind was still in turmoil as I tried to think. I remembered Michael in the general section of the hospital that adjoined the maternity ward where I was. 'Michael, our son, is in the men's ward, Father. He's fifteen. Could he do it?' I ventured.

'I'll see about it!' he said, and left the room, not saying when the baptism was to take place.

Alone again, I thought, 'I must pray!' But I could not concentrate. My mind was racing from one crazy thought to another, as I awaited further information. I still did not know why, and couldn't ask anyone – after all, Sister had said Doctor had to be the one to inform me.

At around nine o'clock, Michael appeared beside my bed in his pyjamas and dressing gown. 'Mum, what's wrong with our baby?' he asked.

'I don't know,' I answered truthfully. 'I have to wait until Doctor comes. Why, how did you know?'

'We just christened her!' he replied. 'We called her Catharine Bridget, I held her hand. Mum, she's black.'

'Black! Christened already!' What did he mean? Keep calm, I told myself. Don't upset him any more – he had to be protected from anxiety because of his ulcer.

A few minutes passed, and we held a guarded conversation before I suggested he went back to bed, promising Dad would come and talk to him when he came later. I needed to be alone to consider what he had said.

How could our baby be black? She wasn't black last night. It cannot be. Dark, maybe, but not black! Even so, she was part of our family. We would still want her to live!

With little concept of time, I saw the other lady return and go to her locker. 'She won't know anything is amiss,' I thought to myself. Just smile and look busy – she is only collecting her toilet bag and will be going for a shower. To my surprise, she came over to me.

'I am so sorry,' she said as she began to cry.

'Why?' I puzzled, what could she know?

'Your baby died, didn't she?'

'Not as far as I know,' was my surprised answer.

Dabbing her eyes, she gathered her towel and bag and left.

Again I was alone with my questions. What was really happening? The hospital grapevine must be running hot with speculation after seeing a priest visit me.

Presently, Noel and our children appeared. After a few minutes of excited greetings, a sister took the children out to see the baby, leaving Noel and me alone. I still had not yet seen our baby since the night before.

'Noel, there's something wrong with the baby,' I told him. 'Doctor wants to see you.'

'I know. I've seen him. He told me she's mongoloid,' he explained, as he tried to contain his emotions.

My immediate reaction is hard to describe. 'Mongoloid.' Momentarily, I could not take it in. Of all the thoughts that had raced through my mind, this hadn't occurred to me. I remained calm. (In control or shock, I am not sure which.)

'Don't worry, it'll be all right. We'll manage.' I tried to console him.

Words seemed futile, and time stood still. The children returned. They had seen their new sister through the glass panel in the nursery door. They were aware something was amiss. I guess one look at their shocked parents confirmed their doubts.

One asked, 'Is there something wrong with our baby, Mum?'

'Yes, there is,' I answered.

'Is she going to die?' came back another.

'She isn't very strong, and we don't know yet. She might,' was all I could offer him.

Their faces were grim but they didn't have much more to say. Before they left, I tried to reassure them that I was fine, and that we had to wait and see what the doctor thought. Those poor kids – their joy had been quickly turned to concern.

Noel visited Michael to try and explain the situation to him. I really don't know how he comforted the family, but I knew it was not easy for him. They spent the visiting hour with me, then set off home.

After they had gone and I was alone, the initial shock was followed by questions, spinning around my head. Why? Why us? How will we cope? We know nothing about mongolism, how can this be properly explained to the children? What will people think? What will this do to us as a family? Our expectations had been dashed! Then came the thought that she might die. Would this be best, as Sister suggested? Again I tried to pray, but I could only hold my beads and, for the first time, I began to cry.

I recall saying to one of the sisters, 'I can't even pray.'

'You are praying,' she assured me.

The sisters had popped in and out at various times during the afternoon. In time, one arrived carrying a baby – our baby. At last, I held her for the first time.

'I'll leave you to get acquainted,' she said, and advised me not to try to feed her, as she had been given some nourishment.

For some time, I just held her in my arms and kissed her forehead. I felt the velvety softness of her skin, and the unmistakable sweet odour of my newborn baby filled me as I looked into her face. She was a dark bluish colour, and I could see the different facial features. I had given birth to her, and she was part of me. My maternal instinct overcame me and, with her warm cheek against my own, I cuddled her close, kissed her soft forehead again and assured her, 'God and I love you, no matter what.' At that moment, I felt a strong desire to take her and protect her from the world.

When it was time for her to be returned to the nursery, I reluctantly handed her over to the nurse. Just then, our doctor came. It was the first time I had spoken to him since the actual birth. He explained that Catharine's colour was caused by her heart being enlarged, preventing her lungs from fully inflating. He didn't anticipate she might live long, but could not really predict what to expect.

Before teatime, I was moved to a private room, which was much easier for us. Michael kept appearing at my bedside and I tried to hide my distress from him. His doctor called on me and asked if I would like him to explain the situation to Michael. I was much relieved, as Dr Rowe had a great bedside manner, and Michael had every confidence in him.

Day 2

My mother rang early in the morning to say how happy she and Dad were for us.

'We're so pleased you have another girl. Maryann must be excited. I suppose you'll be back home in a week or so,' she suggested.

'A little longer, I think, Mum,' I said.

'Oh yes, you'll be needing a good rest,' she agreed, not dreaming there was anything wrong.

I felt uneasy deceiving my parents, but was loath to give her the news over the phone. Both Mum and Dad had heart conditions, and I wanted to be sure they weren't alone when they first heard the real story.

A telegram came from my sister, Mary: 'Crying tears of joy over your wonderful news.'

I was sad for her, knowing how she would feel on hearing the real situation. She was six months pregnant herself, and I wanted to spare her the worry.

On this morning, I did try to breast-feed my little girl, but she wasn't the least bit interested. She seemed to have no suckling instinct, so my efforts were to no avail. Presently, a sister came to see how I was getting on. Seeing that I was having no success, she suggested I might like to try her with a bottle. After trying to force her to swallow, a little at a time, she became very weary – and she had only taken two ounces; barely enough to sustain her, even if taken every two hours. However, after holding and feeding her, I discovered my maternal responses had completely taken over. Her survival had become my focus.

About mid-morning, Noel arrived. He had left the children with a neighbour. We kept our baby with us, noticing her colour had improved significantly.

Noel held her on his knee, her tiny hand in his. 'She's so small,' he said. 'Just look at all that hair.' He began to talk to her, stroking her mop of dark hair.

'Don't get too fond of her, Noel,' I advised. 'You know we're going to lose her.'

We talked about what should be done in the interim. I asked him to place a birth notice in the local newspaper before leaving town – I realised this was something our children would appreciate – and also to ring my brother Jim that night and ask him to go and explain the situation to my parents. Jim and his wife, Pauline, had lost a baby girl at three months of age who had been born disabled some time earlier, so I was sure they would know how to approach Mum and Dad with such sensitive and disturbing news.

Noel spent most of the day with me. I was by now expressing milk and force-feeding every two hours.

Day 3

Noel rang to notify me that our kind neighbours, Mr and Mrs Jack Moran, were bringing Maryann to visit me. I was apprehensive as to what I should say to her, then one of the Mercy nuns who cared for us came in, and I told her my concern.

'Would you like me to talk to Maryann? Perhaps I can explain a little about the baby,' she offered.

'Would you, please?' I replied gratefully.

'Just give me a buzz when your visitors come,' she advised.

An hour or so later they arrived, we exchanged greetings, then I pressed the bell. Within a few minutes, Sister appeared and, after meeting our friends, she asked Maryann to accompany her to the nursery.

Fifteen minutes had passed when a smiling Maryann appeared in the doorway, babe in arms.

I was surprised to say the least. 'Be careful,' I fussed.

'Don't worry, Mum. She's just fine,' Sister assured.

Looking at the joy on Maryann's face as she beamed at the baby, I thought, 'Sister hasn't told her anything.' So I decided to say nothing either.

We had a nice, long visit, then Mrs Moran suggested that they leave and let me rest, before Dad arrived later on. With a kiss and hug, my big girl left me.

On the journey home, Maryann told her friends what Sister Marie Louise had told her. Then to their surprise, instead of the expected tears, she said, 'I don't care – she's my little sister.' To this day, over thirty years later, she has retained that same attitude. There is a special bond between these two girls.

My brother Jim and his wife Pauline, to my surprise and delight, were ushered into my room at two o'clock, having driven one and a half hours from their home. Noel had arrived a little earlier.

'How are you, Bid?' Jim asked as he kissed me fondly.

Pauline hugged me – she was one who surely understood my feelings.

After telling us that they had spoken to Mum and Dad, and conveying their message of comfort and love, Noel took them to the nursery.

Pauline came back ahead of the men. 'Edna,' she said, 'she looks a lot like Leanne. It's just two years since we lost her, you know.'

I didn't realise it had been so long.

Appearing in the doorway just then, Jim said, 'She's our stairway to heaven.'

As we chatted, I told them all I knew about our baby. 'She isn't expected to live – even if she does survive this early stage, she'll very likely succumb to some childhood disease like measles. I might be neglectful on purpose!' I confided in them, as these doubts had plagued my mind.

'Just the opposite,' my big brother assured me. 'Just you wait and see.'

Before returning home, they went with Noel to visit Michael. Between them, it was decided to take Michael to stay with my sister, who lived not far from Jim and Pauline. He could stay with Mary and convalesce until we had adjusted to our predicament. I was much relieved by this, as I knew he would be happy there.

In the days that followed, I had few visitors. Barry and Carmel Mills came one afternoon, while Catharine was still with me after being fed. As we talked, Barry had taken hold of her hand and was looking into her face. He glanced at me, his eyes full of tears.

'You're just like Noel,' I told him.

'It's just not fair,' he said. Barry had been with us and seen our other children grow from babies – he was close to us all.

Father Cosgriff, our parish priest at Bribbaree, called one evening, and we had a long talk. I remember telling him I was concerned about how other children might tease ours. He felt that this wouldn't happen, which proved to be correct. Our children were always so open and positive about Catharine. I guess others followed their lead.

I told Father Cosgriff that Catharine had been baptised. He suggested we bring her to the church at Bribbaree for a special blessing and formal entry into the parish when it suited us.

Judy and Max Curtis came one night. I thanked them for coming – I realised it was not an easy visit to make. I told them of Father Cosgriff's visit, and that he had given me a box of chocolates.

Judy laughingly said, 'Chocolates – you were honoured.'

Father was a very sincere, undemonstrative man – I did appreciate his thoughtful gesture.

Another pleasing occurrence was a card saying, 'Thinking of you', with an appropriate verse. It was from the Bribbaree School Mother's Club, of which I was a member. I realised immediately on opening it just how they felt, and they wanted me to know. I treasured that card and kept it for years, but, after moving house twice, it has unfortunately been lost.

2
Going Home

The doctor and staff were all very supportive and, as they really expected Catharine's death was imminent, advised me to stay in hospital for a few extra days. Even though Noel and our children visited often, I was anxious to take Catharine home, so they could enjoy her for as long as she survived. She was receiving no special treatment and, as John had to return to boarding school in a few days, he would not have the opportunity again. Of course we did not tell the children all of this, because her colour by then was almost normal, and they had come to think that her chances were improving. We did not wish to burden them with our misgivings.

Sister Mary Carr was a very special lady whom I was privileged to have care for me in my years of childbearing. She was now in charge of the nursery and, though most thought I should stay, she was convinced we could manage, whatever the outcome. She reassured me and my doctor of this.

I had been warned Catharine could die at any time – we might just find her dead in her bassinet without prior indication.

Before our release, Sister Carr sat with me and explained the procedure to follow if the worst came to pass. She also invited me to bring baby back to her to be weighed, or any time I needed to talk – just to drop in. This I did from time to time.

When we were to go home, Noel came without the children. Mary and Ron were bringing Michael, and would be there to greet us on our return. With Catharine dressed in her best, Sister Alphonsis carrying her and Noel toting our bags, we proceeded down the hospital hall.

Sister said to us, 'Whatever happens, you must try to treat this little girl as you would a normal child.'

These words often came back to us, and I am sure it was the best advice we could have been given. Thank you, Sister Alfie, wherever you may be.

The chemist was our first port of call, as there were a few items I needed. Noel bought a new camera, as the old one was no longer reliable, and we wanted to have photos to remember this little girl.

Mr Mann greeted us. 'Congratulations. What have we got this time?'

'A girl,' Noel told him.

'Mum must be pleased,' he offered.

Being our family chemist for many years, he was aware we had four boys and one girl previously, but he didn't know of our baby's condition.

'Yes, thank you,' I said.

Another friend – a young man we knew well, John Jarrett, spoke to us at the car. He expressed his concern, and wished us well.

Noel had contacted Father Cossgriff and arranged to have the formal ceremony that same afternoon. This pleased me, as I had hoped to have one of my sisters as godmother, and also it meant that John would be with us.

Arriving home, we were greeted by happy-faced children and a sombre Mary. She did her best to be cheerful, but when we were alone and she was holding Catharine, she said, 'I think I'm going to cry.'

'Go ahead,' I encouraged her. 'We've all done our share of that.'

After lunch, we set off for the church where Father Cosgriff took down all the relevant particulars, blessed, and then confirmed Catharine – a practice carried out when a child is not expected to reach maturity. Father spelt 'Catharine' with an A – an alternative spelling of the Spanish 'Catarina' for Catherine of Sienna. Now when asked, 'With a C or a K?' she explains, 'C. A. T. H. A. R. I. N. E.' with a strong emphasis on the second A.

Michael renewed his pledge as godfather, and Mary as godmother. Many photos were taken with the new camera. Two days later, John returned to boarding school.

In the ensuing time, we were encouraged and uplifted in the knowledge that our family and many friends of all religions were praying for us. We are quite sure it was through the power of those earnest prayers that Catharine survived.

I was producing and expressing plenty of milk, and feeding three-hourly, each feed taking up to an hour to get her to take two ounces or a little more. I had little rest. After a few days, the strain took its toll, and I became nauseous and lethargic. A trip to the doctor resulted in my being put on medication, and I quickly recovered.

Our children were very willing to help – and help they did, in many ways. It is times such as this that one comes to realise just how much children can do if allowed, and how well they understand – much more than they are given credit for, I believe. We were always open to their occasional questions, and answered them honestly. Desiring to give this little girl the best chance, I continued to express milk and store it in the refrigerator. I still harboured the desire to completely breastfeed her, but it was not to be.

Maryann offered to take over the early morning feed, to allow me to get some much needed rest. After supervising a few evening feeds, I agreed. Noel was doing the morning bath time. After all, he was an old hand with babies.

A few days into this program, I was enjoying an extra long sleep-in when I woke to hear Noel's voice.

'Use your finger – mine are too big to clean out those little ears.'

I rose and went to investigate whom he was addressing, arriving unnoticed at the kitchen doorway. I could not believe my eyes – there was Maryann bathing her baby sister, Dad standing by.

'What are you doing?' I asked accusingly.

'Don't panic,' Noel replied. 'She's been doing this for days. You go back to bed.'

There was our ten-year-old, already the little mother; truly capable, and loving it.

Many years passed before Maryann confided the fact that one morning, as she was pouring the last few ounces of the retained breast milk into the small feeding bottle, she knocked the bottle over, spilling its precious contents. Quickly she mopped it up with a cloth, wrung it back into the jug and fed it to Catharine. With her tender years and desire to do the right thing, it wasn't until the milk had been consumed that the fact dawned on her there might have been germs in the cloth. Had she endangered her baby sister's health? She says it haunted her for many months. Each time Catharine showed signs of illness or distress, she worried it was from the contaminated milk.

With her long-kept secret revealed, one of the boys confided one of his own. 'I know it made damned awful Milo.'

Days passed. Always expecting the worst, I watched her closely, and many times I took a peek to check if she was breathing. If, in my anxiety, I envisioned a change of colour, restlessness or heavy breathing, I would secretly take a photo, thinking it might be her last one.

On Sunday, we all attended Mass as usual. Maryann carrying her precious bundle, we proceeded to our usual seat near the front of the church. A friend later told me that there wasn't a dry eye in the church as they watched Maryann and those boys beaming over their baby sister, while they took turns at nursing her.

One difficulty we expected was meeting people for the first time. How would they react? What should we say to put them at ease? Our children had no problem – they had quickly come to accept her as she was, and were anxious to show her off; but I was apprehensive.

Our first social outing was a special parent day at the school. The children had gone to school as usual. We arrived at the playground after lunch. I had Catharine on my lap, dressed in a matching jacket, bonnet and shawl that her Keir grandparents had given to her. As Noel parked the car in the shade of a tree beside the path, other people were arriving also. One couple, Helen and Clive West, came up to our car window and greeted us cheerfully. Helen asked if she could hold the new bub and, as I got out, Jean Schouten followed, stroked Catharine on the cheek and commented on the lovely outfit.

The ice was broken – there was no embarrassment on either side. I will be forever grateful to these special friends. Our children came running up with their classmates, another step on the way towards getting back into the old familiar lifestyle.

3
My Formative Years

Until my marriage, I lived with my parents and five siblings on the family property in a regular, mixed farming district. Mum and Dad were typical, low-income, hard-working people of good character, respected by the community at large.

Both our maternal grandparents were from staunch Irish Catholic background and this was passed on to us. Our dad was Church of England. Consequently, I have always known true ecumenism in practice. Of the children, I was the third, born in 1928 after two boys, Jim and Ron, and followed by another boy, Bill, and two girls – Mary then Janet, who is thirteen years younger than me.

Just one mile from our home was the one-teacher primary school which we all attended. I completed first year, equivalent to what is now year seven. Usually, one moved on after the sixth class. However, I had been allowed to remain and attempt a secondary education by correspondence course, under the guidance of the teacher. I had begun year two when, towards the end of the first term, I became ill with one of my frequent bouts of bronchitis, consequently missing a few weeks of school. I was almost fourteen years old, which was the legal school-leaving age.

After some discussion, Dad and Mum agreed that I should leave school, since Mum needed help with the ever-increasing household chores. Needless to say, I was very pleased, because I was two years older than the sixth class students, and feeling very out of place by then.

Visiting at 'Myrtlevale', our grandparent's home, was always enjoyable – especially at Christmas, Easter or other special family occasions. Many of the families who were able to would gather there. They were memorable days, with love, laughter, music and the unforgettable smell of Grandma's freshly baked bread.

Often, the priest would be there on a Saturday evening before he was to say an early morning Sunday Mass in the little wooden church on the adjoining property. He would drive out from town in his old car and stay overnight. On one such occasion, I recall a joke my uncle 'Blue' played on Grandma. She was busy preparing the evening meal in the lovely old roomy kitchen, when he came in through the back door.

'Gosh, Blue, just look at ye!' Grandma scolded. 'Father will be here soon. Go and get cleaned up and put a coat on.'

'OK,' he responded. Minutes later, he was back. 'This do, Mum?' he teased, as he winked at me.

Grandma turned from the sink to see him standing in the doorway, a wide grin on his face, red hair brushed back, wearing his flannelette pyjama coat buttoned to the neck.

'Get out with ye, ye young devil,' she laughed, brandishing a large wooden spoon.

Uncle Blue was a real torment with a good sense of humour, and it was fun to be around him.

At that time, there was no electricity in rural areas and mothers of families worked extremely hard. The weekly laundry alone was a mammoth task – all done by hand in the wash house, a building set apart from the house. On the wide wooden benches, there were three large, round, heavy-quality galvanised tubs. The largest, which doubled as a bathtub for many years, was for suds in which the soiled clothes were washed.

They were then transferred to the copper in the backyard to be boiled, which removed the remaining stains. Firstly the whites, then light clothes and towels; last of all the men's heavy work clothes. The copper was a large copper bowl set into the top of a forty-four-gallon steel drum converted for the purpose by our father. It was also used to heat bath water, to make soap and to cook yabbies.

On wash day, a large wooden box sat on top of yet another tub on the ground near the copper. This box originally held two four-gallon tins of lighting kerosene which was used to fuel our lamps and lanterns, and was also fashioned by Dad, with holes drilled in the base and hand grips cut into each end.

The boiling clothes were lifted out of the copper using a sturdy pot stick, and placed in the box to drain and cool. The precious water caught in the tub below was then returned to the copper. When cool enough to handle, Mum would carry the heavy box of wet clothes back to the wash house to be rinsed twice – first in clean water, then through water tinted blue with a special blue bag to enhance the whites and brighten the colours. These Reckitts blue bags were small cotton bags containing a block of a soluble blue substance with a cord at the top for dunking in the clear water until the desired tint was achieved. There was a smaller dish, which held the starch – thin, glue-like liquid in which articles were dipped to add varying degrees of crispness when ironed. All these laundered items were wrung out by hand – no mean task for any woman.

I can still picture my small mother with a heavy cotton double sheet draped over her shoulder as she worked along its length, removing excess water. The men's work clothes were also very heavy, as the trousers were of thick worsted cotton, which retained lots of water.

A great improvement came with the advent of a hand-operated washing machine which had a wringer on the top. This appliance was worked by a lever which, when lifted then pressed firmly down, forced a large perforated bell-shaped plunger on to the clothes, pressing the suds through the fabric, removing the grime. The wringer was operated by turning a handle, while feeding the items between the rubber rollers. Again this was hard work but much quicker. My brother, Ron, usually helped with this task.

The clothes line, where the wet items were hung (secured with wooden 'dolly' pegs), consisted of a galvanised wire strung between two poles with a long forked stick propping up the centre, which sagged under the weight of the wet garments.

When dry, the sheets were returned to the beds. The items to be ironed were slightly re-damped and rolled tightly, then placed in a basket lined with towels and left until the following day, to allow the moisture to penetrate evenly. Most household items and clothes were cotton, linen or rayon, and required ironing. There were no synthetic fabrics at that time. I remember when we first had seersucker tablecloths for everyday use, which cut down on the ironing. Later, we were able to buy seersucker fabric for clothing.

Ironing was done on an old woollen blanket, folded on the end of the kitchen table and covered with a double piece of cotton sheeting. Three heavy, flat black 'Mrs Potts' irons sat on the wood burning stove to be used in turn. My aunt had irons with detachable wooden handles, but ours were all one piece, so the handle became very hot as well. To protect our hands, we used a piece of folded flannel, but many burns were suffered. Another piece of flannel was used to wipe each iron as it was taken from the stove to remove any soot. The majority of the ironing consisted of white starched items. A black mark on one of these just would not do, and meant it had to be returned to the wash.

In my late teens, we obtained a petrol iron. It had a small bowl on top into which we poured a cup of shellite, and then pumped air into it. When hot, this produced gas and made a hissing sound. It made ironing much quicker and easier, but I was wary of it. One time I imagined its tone altered, and, fearing an explosion, I raced into the backyard and deposited it there. To my relief, nothing untoward happened.

I well remember a familiar scene in the evenings as the family relaxed, listening to the radio, reading or playing cards. Mum sitting, arms folded, elbows cradled in her hands or rubbing her upper arms. Looking back, I realise just how hard she worked, washing and ironing, along with all the other chores for a family of ten. Dad's parents and brother lived with us. It is no wonder her arms ached. She was a lady of small stature but big-hearted, and I don't recall ever hearing her utter a word of complaint about her lot. She was a truly extraordinary, ordinary wife and mother whose example we, her family, still strive to emulate.

Growing up, I was aware of the accepted behaviour of both genders. My father and grandfather, when working around the farm, used a cart drawn by a draft horse to carry whatever was needed for the day's work. They carried a hoe to cut any Paterson's curse or Bathurst burr if one was spotted. I was forever badgering them to take me along, as my brothers often went, but the reply was always 'It's no place for a little girl!'

Off they would go, perched on the seat of the cart, with a tin of freshly cut sandwiches for lunch, the water bag swinging from the back. I was so envious of those boys.

When I was older, one of my duties each morning was to set up the separator – a machine which separated the cream from the milk as it fed through from the large bowl on top. It was operated by turning a handle at a steady rate – too fast, and the cream was too thick; too slow, and it was too thin. The correct timing was vital. The best result was achieved if done while the milk was still warm, freshly milked from our jersey cows by Dad or one of the boys.

The separator parts had to be washed immediately after use – first rinsed in cold water then hot, then towel dried and, if the weather permitted, left to dry completely in the sun, as all the parts were metal and prone to rust. The cream was used lavishly on porridge, puddings, bread and jam or scones. The remainder was churned into butter, which was another of my chores.

Under my mother's guidance, I first learned to cook my favourite dessert – junket – perfectly set, with a light dusting of nutmeg on top. The aroma was mouth-watering. One day, after the main course of meat and vegetables was eaten, I proudly produced my masterpiece, served with tinned sliced peaches.

'Edna made the junket today!' Mum announced.

My two big brothers and a cousin, Neville, who lived in Sydney and spent the school holidays with us, glanced at each other.

'I thought there was something wrong with it,' one said.

'Sure is!' echoed the other two.

'Take no notice of them,' Mum advised.

But as time passed, there was something I made that they could not resist – it was toffee. After it had been boiled until golden, I poured it into an enamel plate and left it on the kitchen table to cool and harden, insisting it be left until properly set. Enjoying my moment, I would break and dole it out, piece by piece.

One day, Jim, the eldest brother, wanted to try some.

I assured him firmly, 'It isn't hard enough yet.'

'Let's see,' he said. With a closed fist, he thumped into the centre of the plate. Toffee shattered and was strewn over the table. 'Told you it was ready,' he laughed as he gathered up a handful of my precious toffee and left the room.

It seemed that their greatest pleasure was playing pranks on me, and I guess I responded in the desired manner. (Which was their purpose.)

At that time of my life, I could well have done without big brothers and Neville, that red-haired cousin, I was sure. Bill, two years my junior, was my playmate – many a game of marbles, hopscotch or French cricket were contested in the gravelly backyard. Indoors, we would play table tennis or bobs on the large, scrubbed pine dining table. Mary and Janet were too young to join us in play.

A few years later, when I wanted to attend a dance or a tennis match, I was very grateful for my big brothers, as I was allowed to go safely in their care.

On reflection, we had a very stable, happy childhood – growing up with brothers and sisters was a real, character-moulding experience. We have a strong family bond still, even though we all have families of our own.

At busy times, it was my turn to milk the cows and feed the animals as the menfolk took care of the seeding, shearing or harvest. I was also the 'gopher' – responsible for taking food, water bags, the latest cricket score or news on the Miss Australia contest to wherever the men were working. My transport was by horse and sulky or on foot. Brother Jim, being the header driver, had his choice of Miss Australia candidate pinned up on the hessian shade cover that he had erected to keep some of the scorching heat off him during the many long, hot days before the harvest was completed.

Early on, I had hopes of being allowed to go to Forbes, twenty-five miles away, to acquire paid employment and become independent, as some of the girls from our district had done. My dream was to become a nurse. But, like my elder brothers, I was needed at home, and there I stayed until my marriage.

4
'Frankfield'

Until we were married, Noel lived and worked with his father on a grain and wool growing property, 'Wyuna', near Quandialla. He attended the small primary school at Berrendebba, near his home, completing his education at Saint Patrick's College in Goulburn.

At age eighteen, with his father's consent, he joined the RAAF and served four years. When the war ended, Noel volunteered for the Japanese Occupation Force, but his application was not approved. The government saw a great need to return the country to full production quickly, so men from agricultural backgrounds were encouraged to return to farming.

In 1948, Noel applied for and was granted a War Service Loan, which enabled him to buy 'Frankfield' at Bribbaree in New South Wales. On the property was a tumbledown woolshed by the bank of the creek, and a corrugated iron garage beside an old, unlined timber house which comprised four main rooms with a veranda on all sides.

Noel employed a bush carpenter to assist him in making the home liveable. After lining the walls and ceiling with canite wallboard, one room was fitted out for the kitchen. Running water, which I hadn't expected, came from a tap at bucket height beside the stove. The combined bathroom and laundry housed a chip-fuelled bath-water heater and an indoor copper, all of which I had not experienced before.

The main kitchen door opened onto the best part of the building – a ten-foot-wide veranda which was enclosed with timber about three feet up from the floor, and finished with gauze. The floor was well dressed timber, which we oiled and polished – eventually this became our summer living area and a safe playground for our small children.

The renovations were well under way when my parents took me to see what was to be my future home. Mum had packed lunch, which we shared with Noel on the heavy wooden table he had made. As yet, there were no chairs, so we sat on drums with folded wheat bags for cushions. I was delighted with the transformation of the house. I had seen it once in the original state. I was quite prepared to spend the rest of my life there with Noel. Mum and Dad didn't have much to say about the house. Dad was much more interested in the property, with which he was most impressed.

After our marriage, we bought linoleum for the four main rooms which we laid ourselves, with newspaper underneath to protect it from ridges in the timber flooring. A piece left over from the kitchen roll was cut to cover the table. We purchased furniture, an old kerosene-burning refrigerator and a kerosene lamp. With these few items and our wedding presents, our home was complete.

At Christmas, Dad bought us two cane chairs. By our second Christmas, when Michael was six weeks old, we purchased two bridge chairs – our gifts to each other.

Just before John was born, Noel heard of a motor-driven washing machine, which he purchased, telling me that we were adding a little luxury to our lives. But when I exhausted myself trying to get the motor started with no success, I wasn't so sure. It was started with a kick-start, like a motor bike. Noel could start it easily, but I often struggled to get it going.

Noel built pig sties as well as a chook shed and cow bail. After two years, he built a new shearing shed. In all of these projects, I was the offsider. I remember hammering in dozens of nails, and holding many posts and rails in place as he secured them. The early years of our marriage flowed along in an orderly, predictable manner.

Telephones were not easy to get but, towards the end of my pregnancy, in July, we were considered a deserving case and granted permission to have one installed. As we slept on that first night, we were woken by the piercing sound of the ringing phone. Noel sleepily made his way to the living room. The conversation went something like this:

'Hello.'

'Hello. Is that you, Noel?'

'Yes. Who's that?'

'It's Joe. I just rang to ask if you had the phone on. You can go back to bed now,' our jovial neighbour laughed as he hung up the phone.

'Damn Joe,' Noel muttered as he crawled back into bed.

We had employed the services of a seventeen-year-old young man, Barry Mills, in our second year. He lived with us, sleeping in the sleepout on weekdays, returning to his parents home on weekends. Barry was a very cheerful, likeable fellow and an excellent farmhand. He soon became like one of the family. I can remember the summer evenings, with the three of us sitting at the kitchen table cutting up the tomatoes and onions for pickles or chutney, the tears running down our cheeks. We tried all the suggested methods to avoid the sting of the onions, but nothing worked. We all enjoyed the experience, and the finished products were eaten with a feeling of satisfaction.

Noel was a good farmer. The seasons had been reasonable; wheat and wool were valuable commodities and pigs proved to be a good sideline. During our fourth year, Noel began speaking about approaching our bank manager regarding a loan to build a new house. I was sceptical, as we were soon to have electricity through our area. This, I reasoned, was all we needed at present. We were very comfortable, and I knew nothing about borrowing money. I was nervous at the prospect, but Noel was insistent and I trusted his judgement. Soon, we were considering house plans.

As we had two boys, and expected to have more children, it was reasonable to make provision for this. We settled on a plan with four bedrooms, a large living area and veranda on three sides. The local real estate agent, hearing of our intention, called to inform us of a new innovation in home building for which he had just become an agent. It was 'Econo Steel', an all-steel structure, which could be adapted to any house plan and covered with conventional material or another new exterior covering, aluminium, which came in sheets pressed to resemble weatherboards when painted.

With our interest captured, he took us to the property of Mr and Mrs Sid Graham out of Barmedman, where the steel frame had just been used with conventional covering.

Deciding this was for us, since we could carry out much of the initial work ourselves, with eager anticipation we submitted our chosen plans and placed an order, fully aware that this was to be a long-term project. We selected a site for our new home and prepared the foundations under the guidance of a local builder, Ted Tranter.

Within a month, we were informed our order was completed and would be dispatched by rail the following week. Noel and Barry met the train. As soon as the truck carrying our new home was offloaded, they transferred the load and transported it to our site. There were bundles of steel four by twos, crates of aluminium wall sheets with bundles of steel strapping, small hessian bags containing nuts, bolts and washers, plus many other bits and pieces resembling a large Meccano set. Attached to one package were the directions for assembly.

That night, we hurried through tea, put the boys to bed, then spread the instruction sheets over the table to study. We planned to make a start early the next morning, after the usual morning chores were done.

Eventually, between us, with two small boys as 'helpers', all the walls and roof panels were securely bolted together and spread out ready to assemble. Now was the time to recall our carpenter. With Noel and Barry as labourers, and me running food and water, holding things here and there, our home was completed and ready for painting. Two years from start to finish.

By now, Michael was five and a half – old enough for school; John was three and a half, and Maryann three months. It was with much satisfaction at a task well done that we moved in, leaving Barry to sleep in the old house, but to join us for meals.

'Frankfield' was just one mile from the village of Bribbaree, thirty miles from Young, a farming and grazing district. It was the kind of life we were both familiar with and enjoyed, despite requiring hours of hard work and complete dependence on the weather.

During a time of heat and drought, I answered the door to a travelling salesman. He drove a nice car and was dressed in a business suit. I listened to his sales pitch for a few minutes and assured him the goods were very appealing. But, I explained, 'I'm sorry we just cannot afford any.'

Looking around the parched, barren paddocks, he asked, 'Why do you stay here?'

'It's our life, we love it – and yes, country life can be hard in seasons like this, but we can cope, and look forward to better days,' I answered him.

He shook his head, gathered up his goods and drove off in a cloud of dust.

Vincent was only a few weeks old when our first real worry emerged. I guess we were becoming quite complacent, as though we were fully in control of our own destiny. But then the unexpected happened – Noel became ill. After some weeks, he was tentatively diagnosed with a gastric ulcer and advised that he should be admitted to hospital for six weeks of controlled diet and complete rest, the prescribed treatment for this condition at that time. He resisted strongly, but with a wife and five children he loved dearly, he really had no choice. If he was to become well again and take care of us, he had to go.

I had never spent a night in my life without another adult in the house. Barry by now was married and had moved on. Our new man usually came and went each day, but Noel arranged for him to stay in the house with us and went off to hospital content that we would survive his absence. Our protector soon began staying away odd nights. Even though I was nervous, I realised we had to cope. Michael was nine years old and very much a young man, prepared to take over as Mum's support.

I'd had my driver's licence for a few years, but until then had never driven the car to Young, so the prospect of visiting Noel wasn't good. After a week, the children, wishing to see their dad, convinced me I could do it. Choosing a Sunday, when the traffic would be lighter, we set off on our first venture without Dad. I decided it was best not to let Noel know we were coming – after all, he was not to be worried.

The trip took an hour and proceeded without a hitch. After parking the car in front of the hospital, I shepherded my small band of excited youngsters through the hall, led by a nurse who announced, 'Mr Keir, your family have come to visit.'

After much hugging and kissing, baby Vincent was settled down in his basket and Peter climbed in beside his father and slept the whole afternoon away. From then on, we made the trip weekly until Noel was discharged.

In his first few days home, Noel found the noise and activity of his energetic family somewhat overwhelming, following the quiet of the hospital, but soon life was back to normal. From this experience, we learned not to take good health, or indeed anything else, for granted, to count our many blessings and to appreciate every phase of our lives as it unfolded.

We worked hard through good seasons and bad. Our children went through the usual childhood diseases with some prone to frequent bouts of respiratory infections and hospitalisation.

For nineteen years we lived at Frankfield, and perhaps would still be there, but for Catharine's birth.

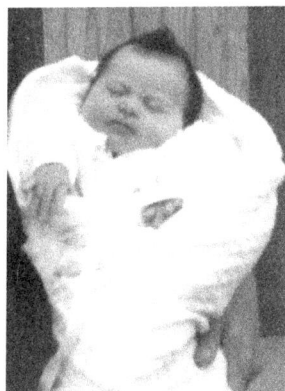

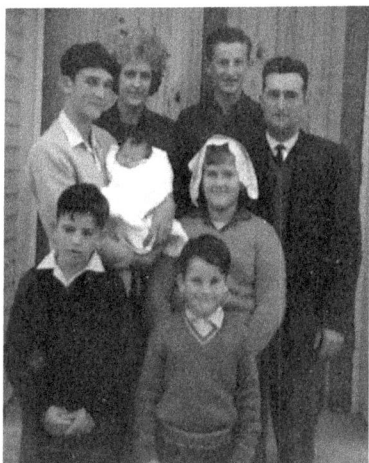

Christening at St Lawrence's Catholic Church, Bribbaree.

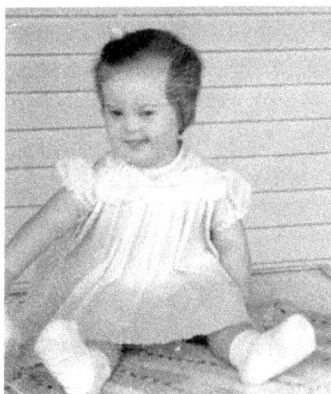

Catharine, 1 year old.

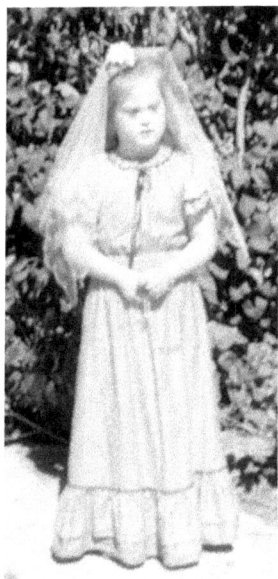

First Communion Day.

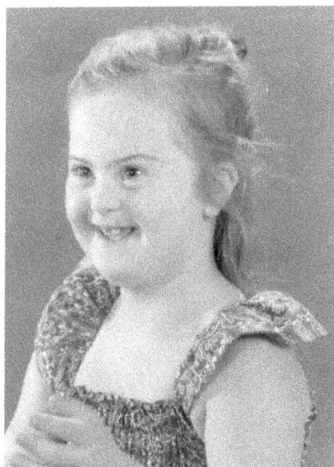

Catharine, 8 years old.

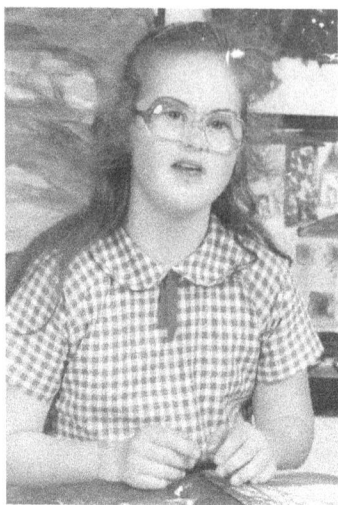

The schoolgirl.

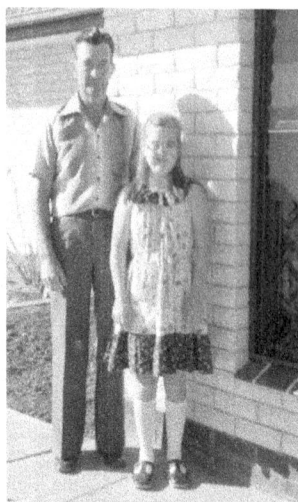

Left: Catharine, 14 years old.

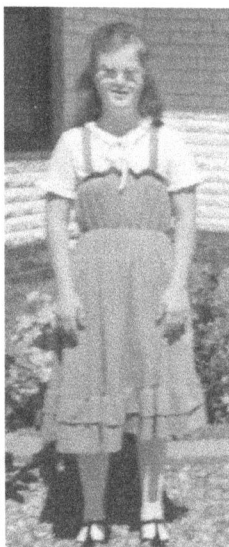

Above: Dad and Catharine.

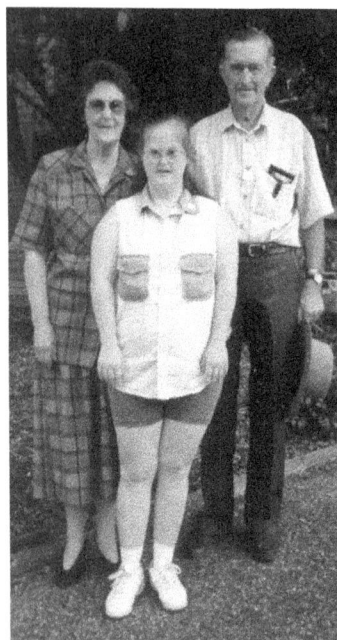

Above: Mum, Catharine and Dad, Newcastle, 1998.

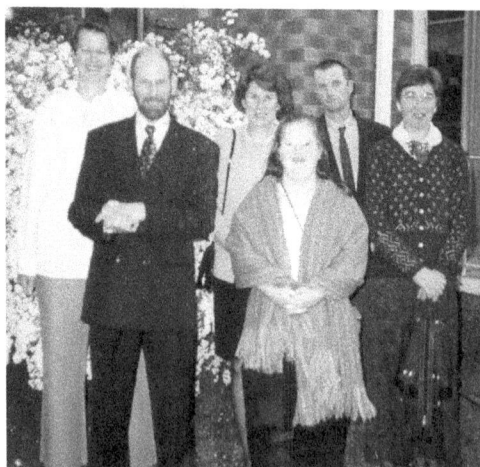

Above: L'Arche household dressed for a formal function, 2001.

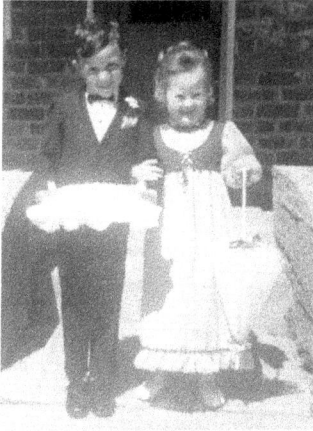

Cousin Gerard Everson and
Catharine at Michael's wedding,
1971.

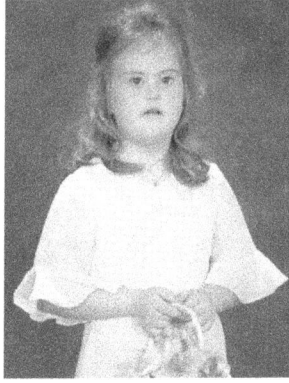

Flower girl at Maryann's
wedding, 1975.

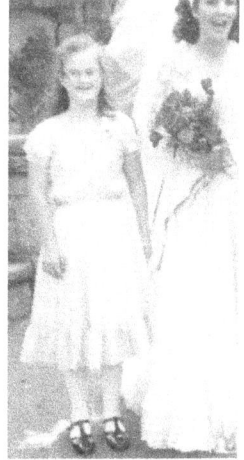

At John's wedding,
1980.

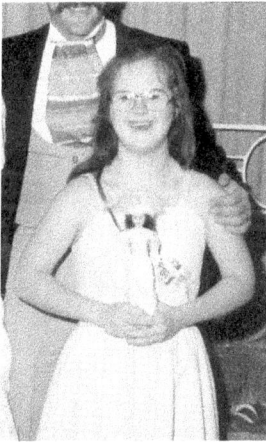

Left: At Peter's
wedding, 1985.

Right: Catharine
and John Peasley at
Vincent's wedding,
1989.

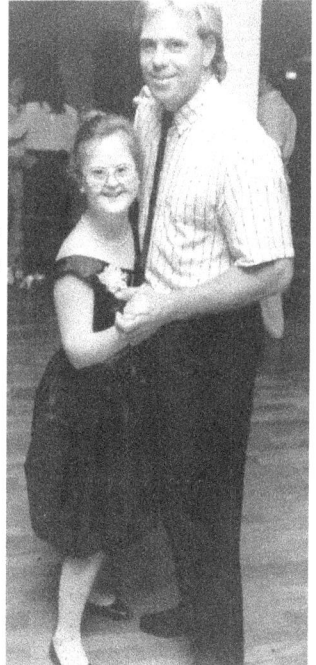

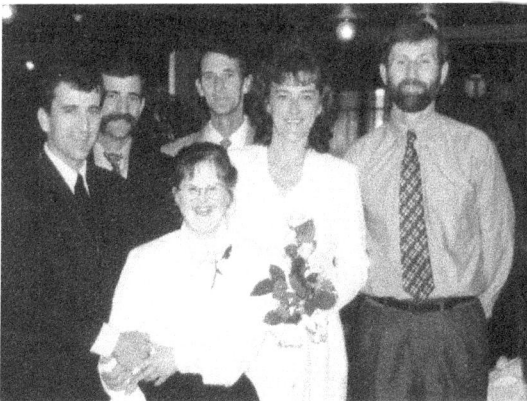

Left: Happy family group at
Maryann and John's wedding,
1994.

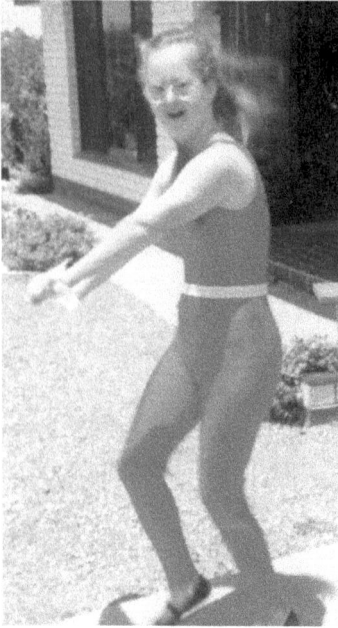
Jazz ballet.

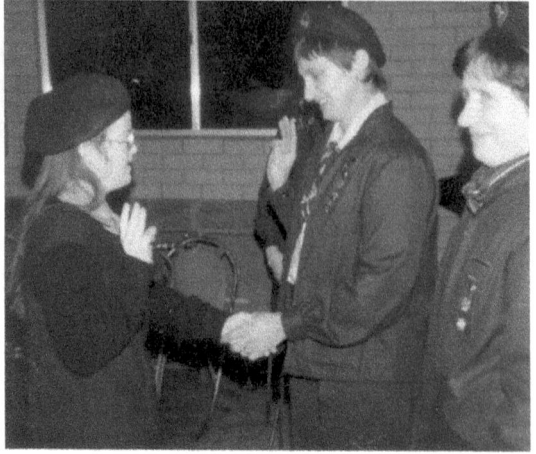
Taking the Girl Guide pledge.

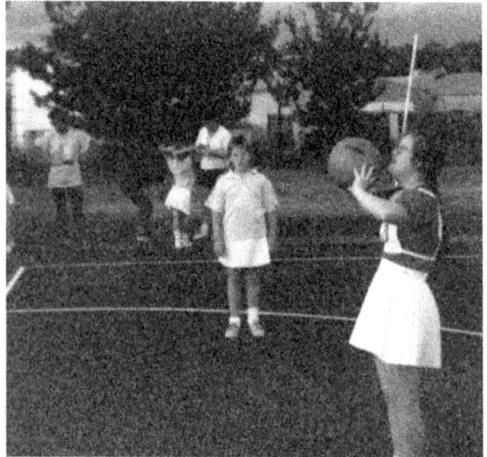
Set to score at netball.

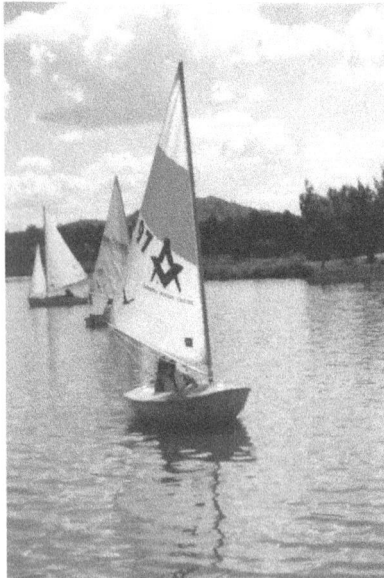
Sailing solo, 2002.

5
Progress

Catharine was a very floppy baby. However, slowly but surely she grew stronger, and did seem to be aware of the world around her. Our love seemed to give her strength.

At three months of age, our doctor suggested we might be interested in consulting a paediatric specialist to have our child assessed and answer any questions we might wish to ask. We gladly seized this opportunity, as we had little idea of what to expect of her, and how to enhance her chances to develop to her fullest potential.

On the appointed day, we travelled to Sydney to see this man who was considered Sydney's leading paediatrician. Our hopes were high.

What help we expected of him I cannot be sure, but it certainly was not what we received.

He looked at Catharine briefly on his examination bench and, after reading our doctor's letter of introduction, he said, 'Yes, she is mongoloid – your doctor knows that. Why did he send you to me?' His gruff attitude did little to put us at ease.

'He suggested that you'd assess her, and advise us on what the correct procedure would be to help her improve,' Noel told him.

The paediatrician looked at Catharine again, this time examining her in more detail. 'There's no evidence of an enlarged heart. However, there is a slight murmur, indicating a small hole in the heart, which will probably worsen as she grows older,' he offered, turning back to us. 'As to her potential, you should hold no ambition for her. She'll be prone to respiratory infection, and at best she may attain the intellect of an eight- to ten-year-old.'

On telling him we lived on a property thirty miles from town and would consider selling and moving closer to where there was a special school, he responded with 'You'd be foolish to uproot your lives that way. If she attended one of those schools, she'd only copy the other children and end up worse than before.' He then advised, 'As she grows older and you need a break, the teacher of the school your children attend might take her for a few hours occasionally.' He appeared uncaring toward us and uninterested in Catharine's future.

We left his rooms feeling that our baby girl's future was very dismal. There had been no encouragement, no mention of early intervention therapy (a new innovation at that time, that we did hear about later). He did suggest we might read a book called *The Child who Never Grew Up*.

On returning home, expecting some help from this book, I placed an order at our newsagent and waited anxiously for it to arrive. I discovered that it was about the author's own Down syndrome daughter, describing how she had placed her in a home for retarded children and how happy she was there. After spending holidays with her mother, this girl was always eager to return 'home' where her friends were. I understood the message he intended to convey, but our baby had a home – ours! – with her own family who loved and wanted her with us. I burned the book and quickly decided the trip to Sydney was of no benefit, except to make us determined to prove this arrogant, high-profile doctor wrong.

The prediction that Catharine's intellectual capacity might reach that of an age ten child heartened us. The experience of our other children was that, at age ten, Maryann was a capable, sensible and dependable young lady and our boys very much young gentlemen, so we could accept that prospect quite happily.

A few months after the Sydney trip, Noel did contact a real estate agent, and we placed our property on the market and began inspecting prospective holdings nearer to towns. Our intention was to give our little daughter every opportunity possible, regardless of the 'expert' opinion – we thought he was wrong!

Catharine did receive 'early intervention therapy' quite unwittingly.

Constantly, these adoring siblings of hers talked to her, nursed, fed and played with her, showing her rattles and toys. They brushed her spiked hair, took her for outings in her pram, and generally stimulated her, none of us realising that what was occurring was exactly what was needed.

Knowing nothing except the gloomy picture we had had painted for us about Down syndrome children, imagine our surprise and delight when she began to flash fleeting smiles around. Our children were elated. It was top news at school. Every little feat she achieved was reported. It seemed that all at the school were interested in this special baby of the Keirs' and had became caught up in the infectious excitement of the proud informants.

Progress was extremely slow, but those kids never gave up – not pushing, but gently coaching, eventually being rewarded with gradual changes that spurred them on.

During October each year, a big event all the family enjoyed was the Bland Rodeo, which took place ten miles from our home. This time I decided to stay home with Catharine, as it was an all-day event. I felt it would be too much for her. With provisions for the day, Noel and the children set off. After feeding Catharine and putting her down in her cot in the sunroom, I lay down on the couch, quickly falling asleep.

Waking some time later, I glanced over to check on Catharine. She was lying on her stomach, gurgling away happily. I rushed over. This baby always slept on her back and never moved. Yet here she was on her stomach. Checking the house, I found there was no one who had turned her over. Could she really have rolled over by herself, I wondered? But yes, she not only had managed it, but also repeated the skilful manoeuvre for the family on their return.

Catharine did not cope well with the heat of summer, so we purchased an evaporative cooler. I would place her nearby in a bouncinette lined with a terry-towelling napkin and a pillow holding up her tiny feet. She was very comfortable, and of course we all enjoyed the respite the cooler afforded, but it was an expense which would not have been considered had we not deemed it necessary for our precious baby girl's well-being.

The sale of our property took over two years. Catharine progressed slowly. At ten months, she began to roll around the floor, before pulling herself along on her stomach at sixteen months, then up on all fours a couple of months later. At two-and-a-half years, she began standing, and took a few shaky steps around the furniture. It was then that we moved house. We were expecting her to take off and walk, but she seemed to lose confidence in her new surroundings and returned to the safety of crawling. As we moved three times within three months, she did not walk until the age of three.

Speech came gradually. With a few words and gestures, she was able to communicate her needs, approval and displeasure quite aptly, and of course the family were quick to react to her every effort.

The shift to our new home was stalled for a few weeks until the previous owner vacated. In the meantime, we moved into a house we had purchased as an investment in the town.

One afternoon, Maryann, now aged thirteen, arrived home from school a little late. She had been shopping and spent her meagre pocket money on a large pink 'My Darling' bib, and announced, 'I think it's time Catharine learned to feed herself.'

I felt a sinking feeling in the pit of my stomach. I knew she was expecting too much this time, and was destined for disappointment. I could not discourage her, so said nothing.

Two weeks later, I was to discover how wrong I had been. The two girls shared a bedroom and, unbeknown to Noel and me, they rose early each morning and, while no one else was around to cause distraction, the lessons began. Vincent and Peter were also in on the secret. By the time her father and I became aware of it, Catharine was eating a poached egg and toast for breakfast by herself. The fact that she would eat an egg at all was contrary to the prediction of the specialist that Down syndrome people have a poor diet – they only eat sweet, sloppy food, and this is the reason they are always overweight.

In light of Maryann's action proving successful, we introduced Catharine to different tastes and consistencies of food, and consequently she acquired acceptance and pleasure for a wide variety of foods.

Because of her slow development, Catharine remained very dependent on us all.

One day, Peter remarked, 'Aren't we lucky to have Catharine? She's still like a baby.'

It took me a long while to stop mentally comparing our little girl with other children of her age. One afternoon when she was just over three years old, Noel and I were sitting on the back step watching her playing in the yard.

I said, 'She'd be lovely at this age, if she were normal.'

He looked at me in surprise, saying, 'She *is* lovely!'

I realised I had put into words what I had been thinking, and felt very guilty. She was a lovely little girl in her own right. This was a turning point for me.

I tended to worry ahead of time, and anticipated potential problems that didn't eventuate. Toilet training was one such issue but, like the feeding lesson, it only took a bit of consistent, gentle persuasion. Menstruation was another concern of mine, but again, with the help of Maryann, who by then was married, plus a program held at her school, Catharine took it in her stride. Maryann still remains her first contact for advice on all 'girl matters'.

Down syndrome people are well known for their affectionate nature. As Catharine progressed, she would respond with outstretched arms to anyone who smiled or spoke to her. This bothered us, and we attempted to modify her behaviour.

Help came from a friend and neighbour, Les Levett, who often called at our home. On one visit, as he was confronted by our impetuous daughter, Les greeted her with an outstretched hand, saying, 'I shake hands with my friends.' He took her hand in his while continuing to speak.

She was captivated by his action. From this instance, we shook hands with people as an example for Catharine to follow while we undertook to establish more socially acceptable manners. Firstly, we needed to educate others who, in their desire to put us at ease when we attempted to restrain her, would react by giving her a hug and saying, 'She's all right.' We were determined, though, and in time, a tolerable level of conduct was accomplished.

Catharine still enjoys cuddles, but now knows when this is acceptable, and offers her hand naturally on most occasions, thanks to our friend Les.

6
'Maimuru'

Our new home, 'Maimaru', was an orchard property, ten miles from Young. It was directly on the school bus run, which was important for our family. The land had originally been part of a large station, resumed and divided into fifty- and sixty-acre blocks designated for soldier settlement after the First World War. The first returned men came from widespread areas and took up residence in 1920. They planted prunes, apples and pears.

The prefab houses were of weatherboard, comprising four rooms and no hall, with verandas front and back. Well before we came to the district, most properties encompassed two of the originals, as one had been deemed not large enough to provide an adequate livelihood.

The main houses were improved to the occupants' requirements, and it was interesting to see the various ways their subsequent owners had done this. The second cottage was invariably left in its original state and used to accommodate itinerant workers during harvest.

There was a mouse plague just as we took up residence, and I shall never forget them getting into everything. We had to contend with mice in beds, drawers, cupboards – just everywhere, for months on end. We found life at 'Maimuru' was very busy, with everyone pitching in at weekends and holidays.

The first crop could not ripen quickly enough. Eventually, a few scattered cherries began to colour and were eaten with relish. Soon, the cherry picking began in earnest. My task was to pack the fruit into cartons for marketing. Following the cherries, we had apricots, peaches, nectarines and plums. The packed fruit was picked up at our shed at 3.30 p.m. by a local carrier and taken to the Young Cool Stores Co-op, where it was loaded onto a large truck to be transported to the markets in Sydney. As this didn't depart until 5.30 p.m., I would take our station wagon loaded with fruit that we had managed to pack after the 3.30 p.m. pick-up, and deliver it in time to be included in the load. Since fruit is extremely perishable, it was imperative that we got it on to that transport. Each afternoon, Catharine and I made the dash to town.

By February, prunes, which were our main crop, had ripened, and harvest began in earnest. This of course was a very different way of life to growing grain, though we soon got into the routine. The first year yielded well, and the harvest ran from mid-November until late March with little time, if indeed any, between varieties.

Noel still had sheep and a modern pig-breeding set-up. Catharine was still toddling when our first fruit season began, and it was quite difficult for me, running back to the house constantly to check on her, or to answer the ever ringing telephone.

The second year, we installed a telephone in the packing shed and brought in a cot and playpen, as I spent a large part of each day there. This was very helpful until Catharine became more adventurous, and tired of the playpen idea. It surprised us all how quickly the little scamp could disappear out of the shed. Looking back, I wonder how I managed, but the reality is, I was younger then. Also, the work had to be done!

Our holding came with its own dehydrator. The prunes, after being gathered, were washed and spread onto mesh trays which were then loaded onto trolleys and wheeled into the dehydrating tunnel to be dried to the optimum level. The heat had to be maintained at an even rate, and was supplied by temperamental oil-fuelled burners which required constant attention.

The aroma and taste of freshly dried prunes is something to be experienced. The drying process, dependent on precise timing and judgement, took some hours. When done, the fruit was removed and, when cold, was taken off the trays and deposited into large wooden crates ready to be transported to the Young Prune Factory, where it was graded and bagged for markets. It became a twenty-four-hour, seven-day-a-week undertaking. Noel set up a stretcher in the shed where he spent most of his time for this crucial period.

As Catharine became more mobile, she loved to get outside, which posed a problem, as the house yard was only partially fenced. One day, she had been playing in the backyard and, on checking to make sure that she was safe, I discovered she had wandered down to the front entrance, just one hundred metres from the house.

'Quickly!' I urged Maryann. 'Run down and get Catharine before she goes out onto the road.'

Maryann dashed out to retrieve her.

'Give her a good smack and scolding so she will learn not to go there again!' I called after her.

Minutes later, they returned to the house, both girls in tears.

'Whatever's wrong?' I enquired.

'I thought she had a nappy on,' sobbed big sister. 'I smacked her too hard.'

'Never mind,' I consoled. 'That's better than not hard enough – she might remember that, and be saved from being hit by a car in the future.'

After a few such episodes, I tired of waiting for a new fence to be erected. I solicited the help of Vincent and Peter. There were some panels of weld mesh down near the shed to be used for future stockyards. With some pulling and pushing and 'Wonder what will Dad say?' we managed to haul up what we needed to secure an adequate area. We wired the panels securely in place, and even added a small gate the boys knew was in the shed. We were quite proud of our handiwork.

On seeing Catharine playing safely in her new playground, Dad agreed it would suffice until he got around to putting up a proper fence. Need I say, it was never replaced and stood for some years, until it was no longer required.

Even though much improved on its original design, our house was dark and uninviting, especially compared to 'Frankfield'. Immediately on moving, we looked at how best to improve the house to cater for our needs. Noel then employed a carpenter to carry out the necessary work.

We reasoned that our need for relocating was much bigger than our need for a grand dwelling. We lived at 'Maimuru' for ten years, soon realising that it isn't the building, but the people, that make a house a happy home, as ours was. We have many fond memories of our time there, and have never regretted our decision to change our lifestyle and location.

7
School

A year after we had settled into our orchard life, we decided it was time to contact Bellhaven School to enquire about the age of enrolment. A friend suggested we have Catharine attend the pre-school in the interim. I rang Mrs Sheedy, the teacher in charge of Bellhaven. She suggested we bring Catharine in soon. We agreed on one afternoon the following week.

Our visit was encouraging. Mrs Sheedy greeted us warmly and introduced us to the students. In no time, Catharine was wandering about, looking at the bright pictures and toys. Mrs Sheedy gave her some to play with; soon she was engrossed in stacking blocks.

'The average age of enrolment has been about eight,' Mrs Sheedy said in answer to my question. 'But it really depends on the individual child.'

I told her of the suggestion of pre-school.

'We have lots of toys and books – perhaps you might consider bringing Catharine here for an hour while you do your shopping and see how she manages.'

I decided to give it a try.

'Tuesday would be a good day for us!' she suggested.

So Tuesday it was.

The first Tuesday, I rushed through my shopping, anxious to get back to check that all was well. Except when in hospital, this was the only occasion Catharine had been left with anyone besides a family member, so I was quite anxious.

On arrival, I found her playing happily. Mrs Sheedy said that she had not spoken a word to anyone. After a few such visits, I became quite relaxed with this arrangement, and was assured that there was 'no need to rush'.

I must confess here that I began to take the opportunity for a little R and R. Really, shopping was not a problem with Catharine – she was quite happy strapped in her stroller or wandering along with a lead attached, but stopping for any length of time was not so easy. What I began to do was buy a magazine, and find a quiet corner in a café to enjoy a leisurely read and cup of tea. Catharine by now was very active, and she needed to be watched every moment, or would quickly disappear. These complete breaks were very welcome and rewarding for me.

One day, Mrs Sheedy told me that Mr and Mrs Herd from the Kurrajong Complex for Disabled Children and Adults at Wagga were coming to speak at Bellhaven, and asked if we would be interested in attending. On the night, Noel and I were warmly welcomed by the local committee, and introduced to other parents who were present. After the main part of the evening, we made ourselves known to the official guests and told our story. They were interested, and invited us to take Catharine to Wagga so they might meet and assess her. They explained that the complex at Wagga comprised a school, workshop and various residential options.

On the morning of our visit to Kurrajong, we were preparing to leave as soon as the children were safely on the school bus. But Michael hadn't appeared.

I went to his room to find him still in bed. 'You'd better get up. We'll be leaving soon,' I urged.

'I'm not going,' he grumbled, 'and if you don't bring Catharine back, I will leave home too!'

'What are you talking about?' I asked in surprise.

'You are going to leave her there, aren't you?' he accused.

'We're doing no such thing. Whatever gave you that idea?'

'Isn't Kurrajong a place where people like Catharine live?' he challenged.

'Well, yes, part of it is. But we're only going so these people can meet Catharine and tell us at what stage she should be able to go to our Bellhaven School,' I explained. 'Mr and Mrs Herd have had years of experience with disabled children and offered their help.'

'All right,' he said. 'But I don't want to go.'

On reflection, I realised we were so busily involved with the business of Catharine's future by then that we had not taken the time to notice the doubt and confusion our other children sometimes suffered.

Our visit to Kurrajong was very pleasant and informative. Catharine was taken into a classroom, and immediately she displayed interest in what the children were doing. Mrs Herd showed her some simple puzzles, and she soon mastered each one.

'Ever since she began to take notice, we've been buying educational toys which the children spent a lot of time and patience helping her learn,' I told Mrs Herd.

'Good work. Keep it up. It has helped and fostered her desire to learn,' she assured us. Then, after a time, she said, 'This young lady is very easy to teach. If you lived in Wagga, we'd enrol her tomorrow.'

'She's only four and a half,' I informed her. 'Bellhaven doesn't take students until much older.'

'With your consent, I'd like to contact Mrs Sheedy and suggest starting Catharine for half a day, three times a week. I'm sure she's ready for her schooling to begin – she's just so keen to learn,' she concluded.

We agreed, respecting her experience in this special field of education.

Not many days had passed before we were making plans regarding which days fitted best with the Bellhaven's existing programs. For the first few weeks, I would deliver and collect Catharine myself, driving ten miles each way. When we were certain she was coping well, and on Mrs Sheedy's advice, we arranged for her to travel on the school bus with her sister and brothers. On arrival at the school they attended, Maryann, with the knowledge and permission of her school principal, would take Catharine to a bus shelter nearby. She would wait with her until a taxi arrived to pick up the Bellhaven students and deliver them safely into the hands of Mrs Sheedy.

The taxi driver, Jack McCabe, also returned the children to the shelter each afternoon, a service he gave voluntarily for some years until government funding provided a free taxi service to all disabled students. Mr McCabe displayed a great rapport with these children, who loved him and their taxi, and we parents were most grateful for his generosity and understanding.

On arrival to collect my little schoolgirl one lunchtime, as was my practice, I found Mrs Sheedy visibly upset.

'Oh, Mrs Keir, I have an admission to make to you,' she began.

I was puzzled, as Catharine stood beside her and obviously had suffered no mishap.

'I lost your little girl today. It was awful,' she continued. 'I have no idea how she got out of the playground. The gate has a childproof clip, and in any case she couldn't reach it. The fence is sound, but during the morning tea break she went missing, and was found across the road at the tennis court where some ladies were playing. I'm so sorry. I watch the children all the time. I just don't know how it happened.'

'Don't worry,' I assured her. 'I know how quickly she can disappear. Come on, let's have a look around.'

On reaching the end of the school, I noticed a wide cement drain under the fence adjacent to the building, not much more than a large cat could squeeze through. 'There,' I said. 'That's where she got out.'

'She couldn't!' Mrs Sheedy protested in disbelief.

'Oh yes she could!' I assured her. 'I know what she's like.'

'The little imp,' she laughed. 'We must see to that immediately.'

'Noel will come and fix it before Catharine's next morning here,' I promised. And he did, making it quite secure.

I collected Catharine at lunchtime until, after a few months, the then president of the Bellhaven committee, Mr John Barton, contacted us to examine the possibility of full-time attendance. This soon occurred, much to our relief – that midday trip to town and back was rather an inconvenience, especially during the busy fruit season.

I must pay tribute to Mrs Sheedy. This special lady was the first teacher of intellectually disabled children at Young. She began quite a number of years before we became aware of the existence of the school, or indeed had the occasion to enquire about such a service. I really can't imagine how she managed on her own for such a long time. She was a truly dedicated lady with no prior experience or formal training in this field. Mrs Sheedy's gentle, caring but firm nature was exactly the requirement for the position she held for some thirteen years. We owe a great debt of gratitude to her – she not only taught our daughter, she also showed us that Catharine was capable of much more than we ever imagined. She helped our girl to reach her utmost potential.

Following her lead, we learned that, by gentle persuasion and repetition, Catharine could achieve so much more, and that, whatever task was set, we must not be prepared to accept less than her best. Until now, we had thought anything she did was great.

I suppose we were still remembering that specialist's gloomy view – but, as for copying others worse than herself, that just did not happen. He was so wrong. I just wonder how many others there were that he treated in the same way, and how many Down syndrome children were cheated, and never given the opportunity to grow because of this widespread attitude.

The first area to which we applied this new precept was speech. Until now, she used more gestures than words and, by responding so readily, we had been unwittingly impeding her growth in vocabulary. To this point, we had found it much easier initially to just go with the flow but, with commitment from the entire family, time and patience, we began to pick up small improvements. We were spurred on to apply the same principle to every facet of her development and it has proven very rewarding over the years.

I must mention here Mrs Sheedy's versatility. Along with the usual reading, writing, and personal care, she taught each student according to his or her particular talents or lack thereof. There was cutting, pasting, sewing cards, basketry, woodwork, tile and matchstick creations, and boxes of all sizes covered with various pictures cut out and pasted on, then finished with lacquer. The quality of the finished items surprised us all, and on open days eager buyers readily snapped up the items.

We consider that one of the most fortunate breaks we have had in our vocation as parents of Catharine was having Mrs Sheedy as her first school teacher. There were other great teachers who followed – they introduced new ideas and skills, but it was Mrs Sheedy who was there to set us on the correct course. By the time Catharine was a little over five years old, she was attending school full time, and continued until the end of her eighteenth year, 1984.

Another first for Catharine came by way of a member of St Mary's branch of the Catholic Women's League – Thelma Millay – who joined Bellhaven as a scripture teacher once weekly. We were astounded when Catharine began to learn The Lord's Prayer. This again was an area we had not yet considered she would grasp, but on which we were jolted into action. From this early beginning, Catharine has developed a strong spirituality and a love of full participation in the Catholic faith of her family. Her understanding of God in her life is quite humbling. Whenever Catharine offers to pray for someone, those people can rest assured that they are prayed for most sincerely.

When Maryann completed her schooling, Peter and Vincent accepted the duty of care for seeing Catharine safely into the taxi.

Brother Dowd related a story to me of how he embarrassed himself, being a new teacher at the school and not aware of our family situation or the ongoing arrangement with the principal. One morning, after class had begun, he glanced out the window and caught sight of the sleeve of a school shirt protruding from the end of the bus shelter. Expecting to find a student playing truant or perhaps having a forbidden cigarette, he walked down. 'What's going on here?' he asked in a firm voice.

'Waiting for my sister's taxi, sir,' came the reply.

On the seat of the shelter, with a small case beside her, sat a small Down syndrome girl, smiling up at him.

'Good lad,' he managed to say in his flurry, and returned to the classroom vowing never to jump to hasty conclusions again.

8
Reading

By age thirteen, Catharine could write beautifully and could spell a few simple words, but her reading skills were limited.

At about this time, Noel and I felt the need of a proper holiday. Our initial plan was to have Catharine stay with Maryann in Canberra, but the special school in her area did not take students short term. A suggestion was made that the hostel for intellectually disabled country children, which had an arrangement with another school, could possibly help us.

Leaving Catharine with strangers did not really appeal to us, but hesitantly we made enquiries at the hostel and were informed that there would be a vacancy at the time we were considering.

She could attend the school, and, importantly, the hostel provided twenty-four-hour supervision. Reassured, we made arrangements – Maryann would be contact person, and we would keep a daily check by phone. A date was set, and off we went to enjoy our holiday in Surfers Paradise.

Maryann duly reported that she had spoken to the supervisor of the hostel a few times, and he had commented, 'Catharine is very happy. What's more, it has been our pleasure to care for her – she's the best mannered child we've cared for in the nine years of our operation.'

This, of course, was great news, and set our minds at ease.

Our return was during school hours, so we were directed to the school before collecting her belongings from the hostel. The headmistress greeted us and showed us into a classroom where the children were settling down in a circle on the floor to hear a story. Our girl among them looked very relaxed. On sighting us, a smile flashed across her face, but she did not move until her teacher invited her to.

'Come and show Mum and Dad around the school, Catharine.'

It was a well set-out complex with a workshop adjoining, where the students graduated according to their individual ability.

After a time, the teacher asked, 'Did you know Catharine can read?'

'Just a few words,' I responded.

'Come with us,' she invited, taking Catharine with her. 'Get your book, Catharine,' She said, and sat us down to observe as they went through the lesson.

To our amazement, Catharine was reading short sentences.

'How could this be?' we wondered – she had only been at this school two weeks. This lady with her special talent and many years of experience with intellectually disabled children had recognised in Catharine her keenness and aptitude. She showed us the method and book used, and encouraged us to take them with us to continue this tried and true method which seemed to be just what fitted Catharine's needs. On returning home, we spent time on it each day, as did her teachers. Catharine's reading improved steadily.

God certainly works in mysterious ways. Had we not taken that holiday, leaving Catharine with strangers, plus the opportunity to have this particular lady's expertise, I believe that Catharine might never have realised her reading potential.

The time came when she was ready to read short stories. This posed a new problem. Most available children's storybooks were more geared for reading to children, not by children, and had been written in America. They often contained names of people and animals that were quite foreign to Catharine. Again, help came from various quarters. Firstly, the small school I had attended, and where my brother's family now are students, was about to upgrade their reading material. The old Red, Green, Brown (David, Sue and Wendy) series were about to be discarded. With Catharine in mind, her Auntie Pauline obtained a full set, and passed them on to us – a real windfall. These proved to be extremely beneficial for a long time. In fact, we still have them, and get them out occasionally.

On moving to live in Young in 1979, we set up as a bed and breakfast provider. One time, a couple from Sydney stayed as weekend guests – the wife was an educator of pre-school teachers, and she became very interested in Catharine, spending time with her and discussing reading material with me.

A week after this visit, Catharine received from our guest a parcel containing two Ladybird readers with a card encouraging her to keep up her reading. So we were introduced to the excellent Ladybird series.

Eventually, our school did acquire a good range of books with more teenage-type stories, simply written. Catharine used these even after leaving school. Her reading skills improved, as did her speech – she eventually was able to recognise and repeat sounds. Even now, we write and sound out words or names she cannot easily pick up.

It has been our experience that intellectually impaired children benefit most from the low pupil-to-teacher ratio of specialised schools, but they generally miss out on the opportunity to mix with 'normal' children. Fortunately, during Catharine's Bellhaven schooldays, a new innovation, initiated by Mrs Dallywater, a teacher at the North Young Public School, resulted in that school inviting the Bellhaven students to attend the infant class assembly once each week. On arrival, our group would be invited to find themselves a seat anywhere. The North Young pupils readily made spaces throughout the room. All joined in show and tell, story time and sing along, then the morning tea break.

Our school was invited to take part in special days, like Book Week and the Easter hat parade. Later, some of our more advanced students joined first and second grade classrooms. This intermingling proved beneficial to the people of both schools. Over the years, many young people have greeted Catharine in the street or shops where they work, calling her by name and enquiring how she is going these days. They invariably are previous students of North Young.

Bellhaven was a private Challenge Foundation school with government subsidy for students until the age of sixteen, at which time they became eligible for the invalid pension. Because these children have the capacity to learn much more, and there was no follow-up facility, the committee extended the school-leaving age until the end of the year a student turned eighteen. Catharine's schooldays ceased in December 1984, and we were faced with a new challenge. Schooldays were the easy times.

Catharine had really just begun to master and enjoy reading when she was required to leave school. We kept on assisting her and were very interested when, in 1986, TAFE offered a limited number of intellectually disabled adults the chance to attend a numeracy and literacy class. Catharine was invited to join the class. She was very keen to attend, as she had an incessant desire to learn and a strong faith in her ability. She did well. The classes were held periodically, and Catharine continued with them up until she left Young, attaining a good level of reading comprehension.

Her interest in food has resulted in a drawer full of recipe books – another source of reading practice. TAFE had also offered various twelve-week classes, one being childcare and the other, basic sewing. Catharine did them all. When, in 1996, she had the chance to be one of the two students offered an evening sewing class for disabled adults, she was very eager.

After two years, under the guidance of their teacher, Catharine Jackson, our talented girl, had made a lovely patchwork quilt for her bed, plus a smart winter appliquéd top and tights outfit for herself. With patient direction, she became quite handy with the sewing machine.

9
Adult Challenges

Our next perceived progress for Catharine was to attend a sheltered workshop of which Noel had been a foundation committee member in 1972. He had held the position of manager for a few months in the early days, during which time he set up the cardboard recycling, and was still an active member on the board of management.

Our expectations were not fulfilled. With the new manager, the board members' responsibility was to oversee the business side of the enterprise, so they had little to do with the daily activities.

It was not until we had a more personal involvement that we discovered how much the workplace had changed under the new government policy of normalisation. Gone were the many volunteers who had happily given their time and talents to assist and teach our disabled adults skills and strategies to enhance their quality of life. They had even acquired contracts from local businesses with a view to part-time employment. Under the new direction, where the goal veered toward moneymaking, the volunteers had been dispensed with, and extra permanent staff taken on.

At our request that Catharine be kept in the building during lunch break, we were positively told, 'She's eighteen. No one has the right to tell her how to spend her free time.'

Our concern was for her safety. Back then, she could not cross the street alone, and had no concept of time. Thankfully, one staff member covertly did watch out for her. Believing she would become accustomed to the workshop regime, we persevered for six months, when a lady who knew Catharine offered her a half-day voluntary position in her private childcare centre. Having had quite a lot of experience by then with her eight nieces and nephews, and knowing how to handle small children sensitively, we agreed it was a great opportunity.

We approached the workshop manager with what we considered a good option for our daughter. After all, the aim of the workshop was for open employment, we imagined – but our suggestion that she go from work at lunch time on Friday to the nearby children's centre did not go down well with him. We insisted this chance was too good to pass up.

Following his ultimatum, 'She attends the workshop full time or not at all!', we reluctantly withdrew her and decided to find other means of occupying her time. This was one of the best decisions we ever made regarding Catharine's future well-being.

The childcare centre trial proved very satisfactory. It wasn't long before she was offered a half a day work experience at another childcare facility also. With references from these ladies, soon Catharine was spending one day doing voluntary work at the pre-school. One grandmother informed us of how pleased she was to find Catharine there on the days she delivered her reluctant, tearful grandson. She said Catharine would take him by the hand and pacify him better than the trained staff. I guessed she had more time for the one-to-one attention he required. Catharine provided assistance at the pre-school for two years.

When a new principal was appointed, things changed. The new principal felt the staff had their own duties and didn't have time to 'oversee' Catharine. As she was in charge, the staff who had previously welcomed Catharine could not intervene.

Catharine's next 'job' was one full day at the new nought-to-five day care centre. Her duties were mostly cleaning lockers, paint pots and toys, but she sometimes read to a restless child or patted one off to sleep. She joined in the music time helping the little ones to clap along, and was paid five dollars a day. This was only one day a week – more was needed.

Noel approached Sister Marie Assunta, the occupational therapist at Mount St Joseph's aged people's home in Young. She agreed to take Catharine one day a week. 'We'll see how she goes,' she said.

We always encouraged Catharine to learn all kinds of craft projects and games. She had also been taught this in school and, when visiting other towns or on holiday, we would seek out craft centres and buy articles for her to copy. This trial was successful, and she began helping out with various craft activities, games and music, as well as assisting with drinks.

Soon she gave up childcare, and was doing two days a week at Mt St Joseph's, continuing until age thirty, when she was asked if she would prefer to join the day care group of her disabled friends who were catered for two days each week. Catharine had previously assisted this group on occasions, but as a voluntary worker was not eligible to join their outings.

This was not an easy decision to make, as it meant she would not have the hands-on involvement with the elderly which she thoroughly enjoyed – but the lure of barbecues and bus trips was inviting. She changed classification and became a day care participant, which she enjoyed until moving to L'Arche in early 1999.

Sport

From early days, our family all played and enjoyed many sporting activities. As we only rented TV during the winter months, the family's leisure time was mainly spent outdoors. Noel had erected a swing in the backyard – it took a long time but, with dedicated persistence by the family, Catharine finally mastered the art of swinging herself, once in motion.

As with most small children, a tricycle was an early Christmas gift, but she just could not get the gist of going forwards – backwards, yes, but not forwards. Then John came home from college on school holidays and succeeded where we had all failed – before the two weeks were up, Catharine was pedalling around the yard all smiles.

Ball skills came quite easily to Catharine. After leaving school, she played netball for two seasons and managed to score a few goals. Also, in indoor cricket, with her ability both to bat and bowl, she was a valuable member of the team. Noel built a wall of marine ply inside our tennis court and bought her a tennis racquet for Christmas. She spent time hitting the tennis ball alone or with others. She was also keen to play soccer with her nephews, as we often watched them in the weekend competition. At the time, there were no girls in the teams, which was a pity, as she would have fitted in quite well.

At home, we had a small pool table and a carpet bowls set – she played both. One day, not long after she left school, we watched a martial arts demonstration.

'I could do that,' she announced.

After constant persistence, I made inquiries with the instructor Jan Smithers.

'Bring her along and give her a try,' Jan suggested.

Needless to say, with Jan's patience and expertise, me sitting through every session taking notes, and Catharine's enthusiasm, slowly but surely the moves began to synchronise. She had attained a yellow belt, then a green tip and was well on the way to a full green belt when Jan moved to another town. We are very proud of her accomplishment, and trust that these lessons in self-defence will stand her in good stead in the future.

In more recent years, Young established a burgeoning croquet club. Noel often suggested I join and take Catharine along. I was reluctant, and resisted the idea. I felt I could not take on another commitment.

Noel, a keen sportsman all his life, still played bowls and tennis. One day, in 1996, he announced, 'Catharine and I are going to learn croquet.'

Which they did. Catharine was warmly welcomed, and offered assistance by the members. With her good ball skills and straight eye, she played 'golf croquet' well, and played each Monday morning until she left Young.

The members of our family are avid followers as well as players of sport. In the football season, each member would claim a certain team to follow, so it isn't surprising that Catharine became a devotee as well.

As we viewed each televised rugby league match, comments flowed freely. Noel was always quick to applaud clean and skilful play. Catharine learned to identify individual players and their numbers. She had her favourites – Wally Lewis always her top choice. In 1989, Wally Lewis visited Young and Catharine was delighted to meet and be photographed with him. Even though she has lived in Canberra for three years, where local patronage is paramount, she remains loyal to her team, the Brisbane Broncos.

Since moving to Canberra, Catharine has played a competitive game of ten pin bowls most Friday nights. Recently, she became a member of Sailability, which is a nationwide organisation dedicated to making sailing available to everyone, regardless of age, ability or physical handicap. We are led to believe that she is fast becoming a proficient solo sailor, and she has recently competed in an international regatta at Canberra.

10
Friends and Frustrations

Over the years there have been numerous painful incidents – we have all had to deal with them even though the hurt is always there. It has been gratifying to Noel and me to watch our children grow and mature in this quite difficult area for siblings and parents alike.

From the very beginning, our children were eager to talk about their sister to anyone in their own way, and generally the result was positive. I assume as children they were not too preoccupied with her classification – to them she was just Catharine. Friends were all interested and supportive. As the years rolled on, children became teenagers, friends likewise, boyfriends and girlfriends came and went with never a hint of a problem. In fact, everyone seemed to have a place in their hearts for this little girl, with her affectionate nature and ready smile. As a family, we did insist on a certain amount of discipline for her, and unacceptable behaviour was not tolerated.

One evening, Catharine and I were singing along with people at the retirement village. It was an annual Christmas concert to which people who had been involved in entertaining the residents throughout the year were invited. Seated close by were three children from one family. They were very talented singers who often performed in public. Having already presented their item, the trio sat with their accompanist. Instead of joining with everyone else, they were engaged in tittering at Catharine, who, quite oblivious of their amused attention, was doing her best to sing the Christmas carols she enjoyed. Their pianist, a lady I knew, sensing I had noticed, gave me an embarrassed smile. I considered this event for a few days and decided to contact their school principal, to whom I related the story. I asked if children at the school were not taught basic manners and that whatever talents we have are gifts from God to be thankful for – that all people are God's creation, with or without obvious endowment, and deserve respect.

'Even Catharine, whom these children consider a joke, feels hurt when stared at, and knows not to stare or be disrespectful to others herself,' I concluded.

The outcome of this visit was a suggestion that I might give a talk to years seven and eight on disabled people. I was not confident in my ability to do it well, but did accept the invitation.

I carefully prepared notes on what I considered appropriate. On the appointed afternoon, I passed the church on route to the classroom. I went inside and knelt in front of Our Lady's altar and prayed. 'You of all people understand my plight. Your own child was not always treated kindly, was often laughed and jeered at. Please pray to God that His guiding hand be on me in this endeavour.'

Minutes later, I stood at the front of the class. I was aware of a sea of faces as the teacher introduced me. I opened my notes, and the time passed quickly. Questions and comments came freely.

At the end of the allotted time, the teacher called a halt, thanked me and, as I prepared to leave, said, 'Don't lose your notes, Mrs Keir. We may call on you again some time.'

It was then that it dawned on me. I had not followed my notes – the guidance I had prayed for had been granted. I returned to the church to give thanks.

Soon after we moved to 'Maimuru', while attending Mass at St Mary's Church, Young, we sat near the front of the church as was our custom. Maryann held Catharine, then aged three, during the homily. Catharine brushed her foot against the lady in front of her, who glanced around. Catharine enjoyed the attention. Moments later, she reached out her foot and touched the lady's back again. Immediately, this well dressed lady turned and glared at both girls, who responded with smiles as Maryann tucked the offending feet back in firmly.

In my then fragile state, I was very hurt, and tears welled in my eyes.

'What's her concern?' I brooded. 'Even if she had her expensive coat soiled, all she need do is have it dry-cleaned. Our "problem" is permanent.'

At this time, Catharine wasn't yet walking – her shoes had never touched the floor, let alone become dirty. I had hoped the glare had passed unnoticed by all but me. But on the way home John remarked, 'That lady didn't like Catharine touching her coat, did she?'

Not wishing to pass on my own reaction, I did some quick thinking. 'I suppose she thought her shoes were dirty,' I defended her reluctantly, hiding my hurt. Looking back, it was a gross overreaction on my part, but it did happen.

Another time a couple of years later, the primary school both Peter and Vincent attended was hosting visiting city school sports teams to a barbecue in the park. As parents, we were assisting. Noel was at the barbecue and I was buttering bread, with Catharine playing happily near by.

'OK, folks,' came from the teacher in charge. 'Line up, food's ready.'

After a time, I realised Vincent had not passed along for his meal. Looking around, I spotted Peter and asked, 'Where's Vincent? He hasn't had his lunch.'

'In the car, I think,' he said.

'Is he sick?'

'Don't think so,' he answered guardedly.

I gathered Catharine up and went to the car to find Vincent there by himself. This was out of character for this sociable young lad who enjoyed being in the middle of the action with his mates. He appeared quite dejected.

'What's up?' I enquired. 'Are you sick?'

'Nuh!' was the reply.

'Come on, then. The sausages'll soon be all eaten. You'll miss out.'

'Nuh. Don't want any!'

'Why? You must be hungry.'

Again, 'Nuh.'

'Come on,' I coaxed.

'No. I want to stay here.' He was adamant.

What could be wrong, I puzzled, realising that something had upset him and he did not want to tell me.

'Have you had a fight?'

But he was non-committal. After some time, he reluctantly opened up. 'Some city kids are talking about Catharine. One said she had a flat face.'

For a few seconds I said nothing. What could I say? He was so hurt at this affront to his beloved little sister. 'It's all right,' I tried to explain. 'They don't know her, and don't mean any harm. You know what kids are like.' I rattled on, groping for words to help him, not wanting to condemn the boys who had caused his anguish. I persuaded him to rejoin his friends.

Of course, there have also been happy and positive reactions. It became my practice to shop one afternoon a week at Favero's Supermarket. The three schoolchildren would meet us there after school. With Catharine sitting happily in the shopping trolley eating a small packet of chips, I trundled up and down the aisles, scanning the shelves. When the children arrived, she greeted them – all smiles, and arms outstretched. Lifting her out, they would hug and kiss her in turn, she insisting on sharing the crumbs in the bottom of her chip bag with them.

Tony Favero, one of the sons who worked in the family business, commented to me one afternoon, 'It's the highlight of my week when your kids come, the way they greet Catharine with such open and genuine affection. It's rare to see big boys like them show their true feelings in public with no hesitation at all.'

I thanked him for his remarks, thinking to myself, 'Aren't all families like this?'

In 1970, John was seventeen and still at St Patrick's College, Goulburn. The annual open weekend was being held. Noel and I decided to go and surprise him. So, with the family, we drove down, arriving just as everyone was settling on seats outdoors for the official opening ceremony. We found a vacant stool near the back and sat down to listen. Soon I recognised John's back just a few rows in front of us sitting with a young lady friend.

I whispered to Catharine, 'There's John!' and pointed him out to her.

Minutes later, she slid off my knee and silently wended her way through the chairs until she stood beside her big brother.

On seeing her, John whispered to his companion, 'There's a little girl like my sister Catharine.' Then, 'It *is* Catharine!' he said in disbelief, as she scrambled onto his knee. Glancing around, he spotted us and smiled, but he had to stay for the time being with Catharine firmly planted on his knee until the formalities were over.

Until about the age of eight, Catharine was prone to respiratory infections, as had been predicted, and was hospitalised in the Mercy Hospital a few times. On one of these occasions, when she was five years old, Michael would call to see her on his way through town to visit his girlfriend (now wife), who lived at Harden.

One day, a lady stopped me in the street and introduced herself. 'I'm Kay Waugh. We haven't met, but I know you're Mrs Keir! I just wanted to tell you how impressed I've been with your son.'

'Yes, I'm Edna Keir. Which one do you mean? We have four sons.'

'He's about nineteen or twenty, I guess – tall and dark,' she explained.

'That would be Michael, our eldest. Where did you meet him?'

'I didn't really meet him, but I have seen him visiting his little sister in the Mercy some evenings while I've been sitting with my daughter – she was in with a broken leg at the same time as your little girl. It was just beautiful to see him with her, and her delight on seeing him walk in – her arms shot up, and he'd lift her out of the cot. She'd then wrap her arms around his neck and kiss him. After a time, he'd proceed to brush her hair and put it up in a band, all the while carrying on a bright conversation, quite oblivious of others around the room. My eyes just filled with tears, he's so lovely with her,' she concluded.

'Thank you, it was nice of you to tell me,' I said as we parted. The frustrations were always tempered with moments like these.

I must explain the hairband situation. Catharine had silky straight hair which fell all over her face if not tied up. I could well visualise Michael replacing the band, as it was impossible to keep it in place for any length of time. The entire family hated to see her hair in her eyes, and became adept in this procedure.

We were also given the gift of really good friends who helped along the way. Ken and Valerie Moran, who were neighbours at Bribbaree and who also moved to Young, were always encouraging us to do a coach tour. They had been on many coach and caravanning trips since their family had all married. We agreed that this would be nice, but not very likely.

They persisted, however, and Val offered to take Catharine for a month while we travelled, saying, 'There's a tour at the end of July. We've done the trip and I'm sure it would suit you!'

We were non-committal.

'Catharine will be fine with us,' Val insisted. 'Think about it!'

It seemed too good to be true, and we discussed it for days before deciding to accept their generous offer.

We returned from this wonderful Queensland holiday to find our girl happily ensconced in the Moran household!

Another time when our treasured friends stepped in was when Noel had been hospitalised in Canberra for surgery. Noel and Mary Moloney took Catharine into their home, leaving me free to be with my husband when he needed my support. We are most grateful to these special people for their practical and thoughtful assistance.

Things that go unnoticed by the general public can be quite arduous to families like ours. It wasn't until we first attempted to teach Catharine to read basic, vital signs like Stop and Go, Hot and Cold, Danger, Wet Paint and others (also identifying which toilet to use) that we became conscious of the many and varied words and symbols used. For example, ladies, gents, lads, lassies, women, men, girls, boys, guys, dolls, colts, fillies and some dubious features and caricatures of animals and birds – believe me, we saw them all.

These frustrations became ongoing and had to be dealt with constantly. This proved very confusing for a small girl with intellectual difficulties, and just another dilemma for her family to deal with. I guess we were looked on somewhat as curios while we went through our rituals, wherever we happened to be. Again, with unified persistence, we did what was required, no matter the circumstances, until the desired result was achieved.

In the early years, Catharine's speech came haltingly – just broken sentences, omitting many connecting words. For instance, 'Kids school?' meant 'Are the kids at school?'; 'Dad work?' – 'Is Dad at work?'; 'Church?' – 'Are we going to church?'

Catharine and I spent many twenty-minute trips to and from town for various reasons. I used the time to teach her to use full phrases. In the beginning, we used nursery rhymes – as she loved music, it was more enjoyable for her if we sang.

Baa Baa Black Sheep began as 'Black Sheep Any Wool'. Mary Had a Little Lamb was 'Mary Lamb'. Then there was 'Jack Jill Hill' and others. We never gave up, and she gradually began to retain one-liners.

There were some words Catharine could not pronounce, which I believe is quite usual for Down syndrome people.

Eventually, after she had been at school a few years, I made enquiries about speech therapy, only to be informed by the community health centre that speech therapists were not trained to deal with intellectually handicapped children. After some perseverance, we were given an appointment with a therapist who visited Young from Canberra twice a month. This young lady indeed had no experience in our field, but began by teaching me the basic routine of encouraging Catharine to watch my mouth closely as I formed words, then to get her to watch her own mouth in a mirror as she endeavoured to voice the same words. After a few visits, I was able to continue alone. You can imagine that this was an exacting and painstaking process. Gradually, her speech became more easily understood.

Some years later, we were able to access a resident therapist at the local health centre to assist with sounds we still had difficulty with. This therapist suggested we use a tape recorder to record Catharine's speech and play it back to her – and a very useful tool it proved to be. This has been an ongoing process. Consequently, Catharine's speech is very good for a Down syndrome person. As she loves to converse with people, we have always impressed on her the importance of correct pronunciation, which continues to improve with much repetition, and with her reading ability.

I recall my father once commenting, 'Maryann is happiest when she's doing something for someone else.'

This is a characteristic her sister shares. Being a late riser, I have often been the recipient of their attention, being served tea and toast in bed and other special treats.

I was fifty-nine and had not played tennis for a few years when I teamed up with Maryann for a night tennis competition. The morning after our first match, I woke extremely stiff and sore and decided to take a long soak in a hot bath. I shuffled towards the bathroom, trying not to move a single muscle. As I passed Catharine, I said to her, 'If anyone rings and wants me, I'll be in the bath for a while.'

'Are you all right?' she asked anxiously.

'I will be!' I assured her.

I had just begun to relax in the soothing water when a gentle knock came on the door. I heard a softly spoken 'Can I come in?'

'Yes. What do you want?' I muttered, not wishing to be disturbed.

The door slowly opened. There stood Catharine, tray in hand. 'I brought you breakfast,' she explained.

'You spoil me,' I said as I took the tray. I felt totally indulged, and wondered how many others enjoy such luxurious attention.

11
Weddings

Michael's wedding was the first of five. I was hesitant when Lou asked if Catharine, aged five, could be the flower girl. They explained that Gerard, Catharine's cousin of the same age, had been asked to be pageboy. I agreed, knowing he would lead her. There was a rehearsal the evening before the wedding. Early the next morning, the bridesmaids, flower girl and I set off for the hairdresser. This was Catharine's first professional hairdo.

Her long hair was set in curlers like the rest of us, but she would not have the hairdryer over her head, no matter how we coaxed. Mary Silk, who was doing our hair, suggested we leave the rollers in to dry naturally and call at her house on the way to the wedding to have it combed and pinned up. We did this, and Mary did a beautiful job. The hair looked just lovely and the curls lasted throughout the entire evening.

It was a wonderful family day. The two girls were bridesmaid and flower girl along with Lou's sister and a friend. John was groomsman; Peter and Vincent assisted the priest for the mass as altar servers. The tiny flower girl carried out her duties with great aplomb and pleasure.

John's career path had led him to Sydney directly from college, but Michael lived and worked from home, as did Maryann and Peter after their schooldays were complete. Vincent took up a career in nursing.

Michael's means of transport was a cream Dodge utility with the muffler adjusted to produce the desired sound, befitting a young man of the time. It was quite distinctive and readily recognised as he drove over the ramp at our front entrance and up the drive. A few days after he and Lou were married, Catharine was sitting on the kitchen floor, her back against the door of the deep freezer. The motor jumped into gear with a loud throbbing sound.

'Michael, Michael,' she called, as she sprung to her feet and dashed out the door, only to be disappointed. She had been missing him and was excited to hear what she thought was his vehicle coming up our drive.

Our next wedding was Maryann's. By then, Catharine was almost ten years old, and was very interested and involved as the event drew near. I had driven the girls to Wagga to select and order frocks and accessories a few weeks before the chosen date. The excitement increased as each parcel arrived and its contents were revealed.

Again, the wedding was a family affair. John and Peter drove the bridal cars, Catharine was the flower girl, Vincent was the vocalist and Michael was master of ceremonies at the reception. The day went well but, because these sisters have a special bond, all were a little anxious about how Catharine would react to Maryann leaving the reception. When the ceremonies were over, after changing out of her wedding frock, the bride and groom returned to say their farewells.

Catharine was playing and dancing in the centre of the hall as we took our places in a circle. Maryann went straight to her, crouched down, took her hands in her own and engaged in earnest conversation for quite some time. With a kiss and hug, the sisters parted all smiles, but there were a few damp eyes around the room. Whatever was said was all that was necessary.

On their first visit home after settling into their unit in Canberra, Maryann informed us that she wanted to take Catharine back to Canberra for a week, the reason being to acquaint Catharine with where she was now living, to allay any doubts or fears she might be harbouring about losing contact.

'That's a lot to expect of Don,' Dad suggested.

'Dad, we've discussed this, and Don agrees,' he was told.

On returning home a week later, Catharine was all talk about Maryann's house, quite happy in the knowledge of where her big sister was and that we could see her often. Noel and I were again to acknowledge the thoughtfulness and wisdom of our young people.

John and Janine were married a few years later and, in due course, Peter and De'hanne, then Vincent and Sue. Though not in the bridal parties,

Catharine received her own official invitation, and became caught up in the excitement of each wedding. Together with Mum, there was always a new dress and shoes to be purchased and, as a special touch, a shoulder posy.

Catharine has always been accepted and made to feel as important as every other member of the family. She is expected to behave as a responsible adult – she has no difficulty with this. From the very beginning, it was agreed that Catharine must be disciplined, which wasn't easy with her limited intellect early on, but, again, combined persistence paid off.

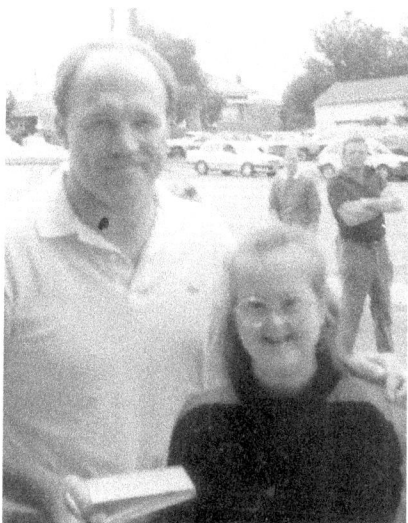
With Wally Lewis at Young, 1989.

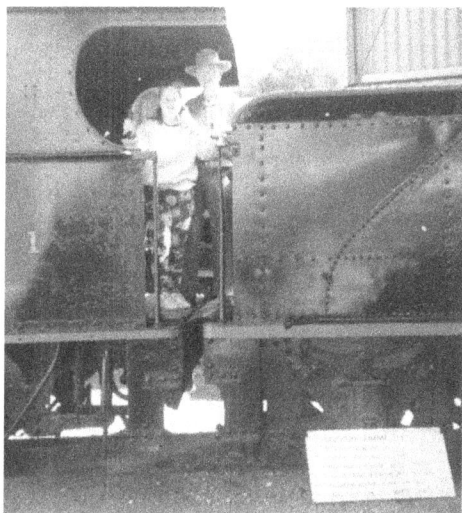
Dad and Catharine at the Railway Museum, Broken Hill, 1996.

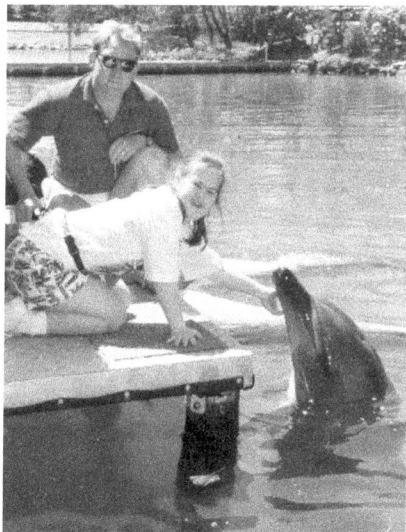
A friendly dolphin, Seaworld, Surfers Paradise.

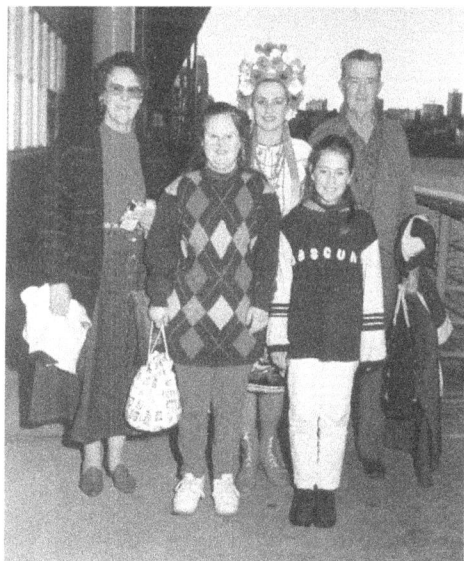
Mum, Catharine, Keren and Dad with the hostess, boarding the Karelia, *1999.*

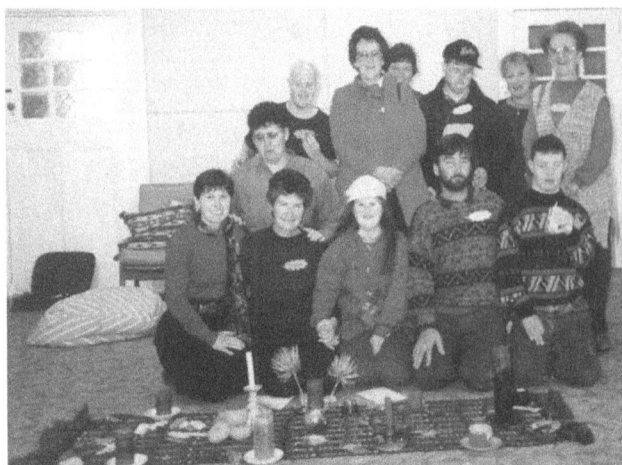

Faith and Light.
Top: Galong, 1995.
Centre: Albury, 1999.
Bottom: Lourdes, 2001.

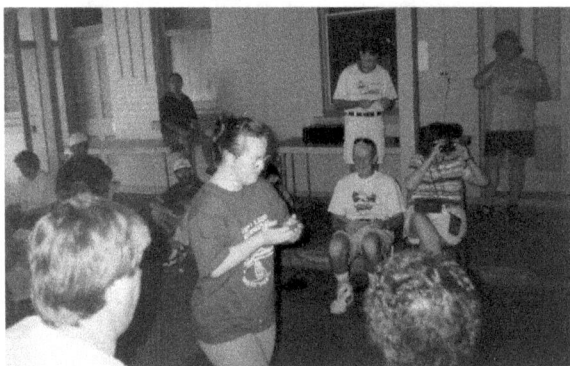

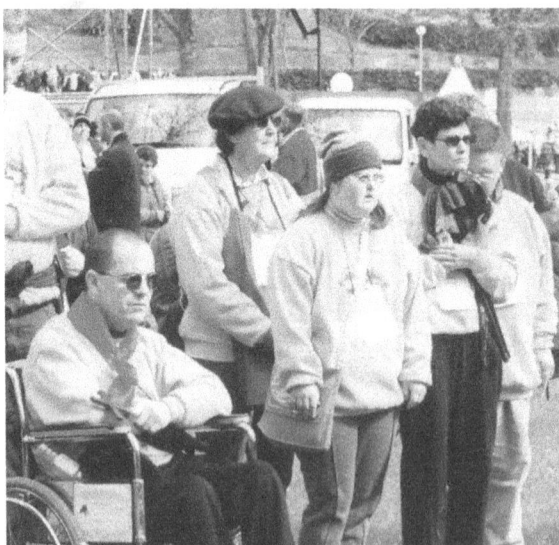

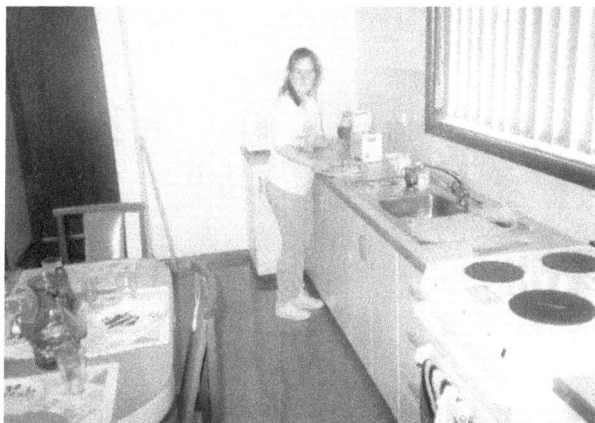

Left: Catharine in her new kitchen, 1992.

Right: Kaleen and Catharine at home, 2002.

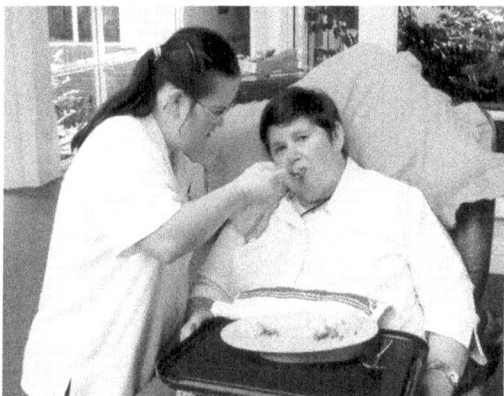

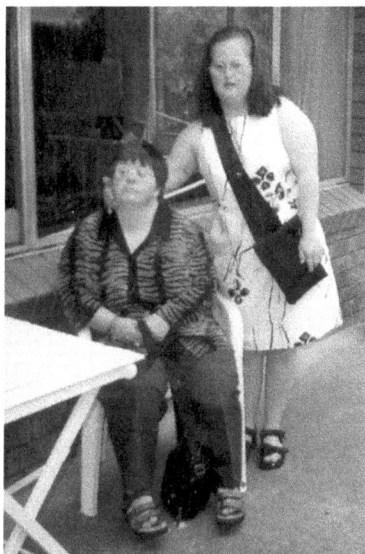

Above and right: Catharine as volunteer at the aged care centre, 2003.

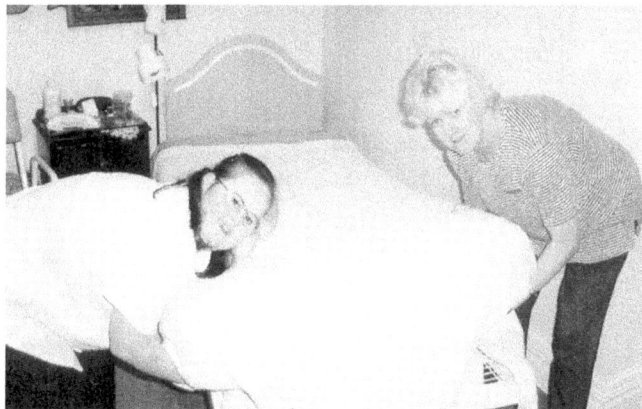

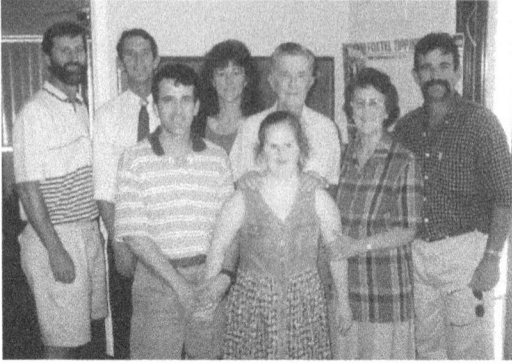

Last family group with Dad, March 1998.

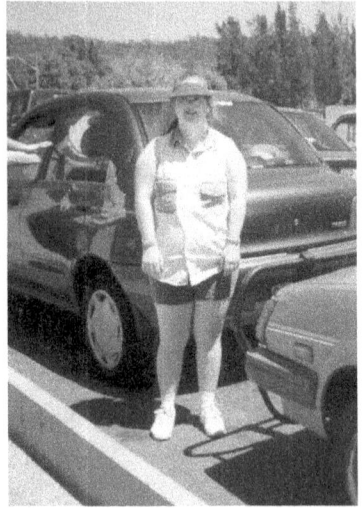

On the Wiseman's Ferry, 1998.

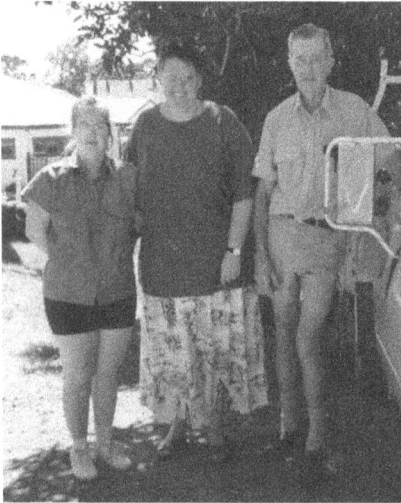

With Sr Joanne at Lawson, 1998.

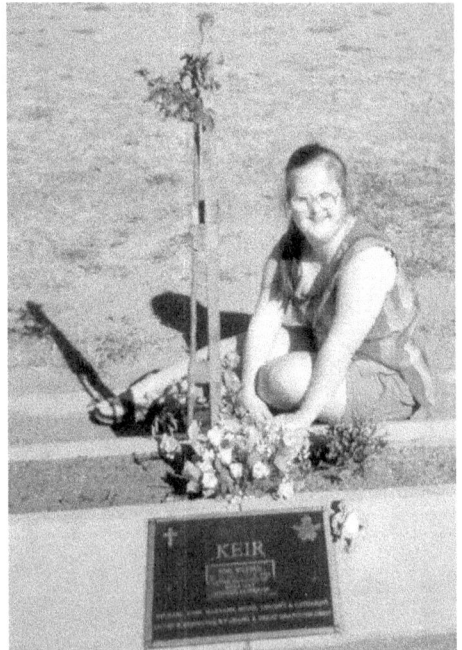

Dad's grave complete with angel, 2000.

12
Our New Ventures

In 1972, Noel reasoned that because we had such a variety of fruit in the summer and plenty of land to produce vegetables, we might consider purchasing a greengrocery shop that was being advertised for sale in Young. After inspecting the business, a deal was done and we began a new venture.

Michael and I became the shopkeepers. Later on, we employed part-time staff. I had never worked behind a counter before, but soon became accustomed to it. Maryann was working in town, Peter and Vincent were still at school. Catharine would be dropped by taxi at the shop to travel home with me. Our family learned a great deal by taking their turn serving customers – even though the customer is always right, believe me, sometimes they could be very difficult. We kept the shop for four years. By then, Maryann was married, Peter was working and Vincent was at boarding school.

In 1979, we sold the orchard and bought an eleven-acre block in town. This was part of a property that had been developed around the boundary – a perfect spot for us, just fifteen minutes walk from the centre of town. We built a four-bedroom brick-veneer home and settled in. Catharine and I revelled in town life, and we were able to give her many more opportunities. I became her 'taxi' as her social life blossomed. Peter was still living at home, but Vincent had moved to Sydney by this time.

Noel's aversion to retirement resulted in him purchasing two hundred acres of land five miles from town, on which he set up angora goat breeding. This was new to us but, with Noel's ambition to try new challenges, he became very involved and gained much pleasure from it. Eventually, he sold the land and kept a few of the top-grade does here in the town area, from which he continued to breed for a few years.

The fluffy white kids were most entertaining as they frolicked over the rocks and logs. I learned to spin the hair, and then knitted garments for all the family from the silky white yarn. I sometimes blended it with wool from coloured sheep to give the fibre special tints and texture.

As Noel thoroughly enjoyed being with people, he took a position at the Gas Pipeline Authority, and continued to hold the contract as groundskeeper for eight years. This was a large area with lawns, trees and shrubs. Noel made many friends there, and Catharine and I were often included in staff social events. The Christmas party was great, highlighted by the arrival of Santa, in their helicopter.

In 1989, after attending the first Down syndrome conference, Noel was very eager to give Catharine the chance to experience independence by having her own quarters. I was hesitant – I could picture myself running backwards and forwards, keeping two homes in order. But I had to admit it would be great for Catharine if it worked out.

During the next twelve months, we looked at a few options. The best one seemed to be to build a self-contained flat onto our house, encompassing an existing bedroom. Catharine moved in at Christmas in 1991. The entire family came to make it a real house-warming with many gifts.

Catharine took to her own quarters readily, and was soon living independently except for the evening meal, which was mostly eaten with us. As time passed, Catharine enjoyed her privacy more and more. She took up new crafts, and became adept in long-stitch pictures and hooked floor rugs. We thought we might find someone to live with Catharine, but this never came to be. She did enjoy having her own visitors occasionally, becoming quite the hostess at every possible occasion.

Recently, I asked my family what they remembered about Catharine's earliest days. The general consensus was 'Mum needed a lot of help and care.'

What a burden to put onto young children and their father, who were confused and hurting. They had been made to feel responsible for my welfare by misguided advice from well-meaning people! By being unaware of this, I did nothing to alleviate their concerns for me.

Is it the same today? I fear, yes – the mothers are surrounded with sympathetic support whilst the dads are expected to cop it on the chin and get on with things.

In the eighties, there was a mothers of disabled group at Young. It afforded mothers great solace. The realisation that others had identical anxieties and insecurities resulted in a healing process for many of us, who shared our stories and experiences over a cup of coffee.

I suggested there should be a similar group for fathers, but it did not eventuate. This attitude of 'He's tough, he'll be OK' towards dads is regrettable and the cause of some fathers feeling excluded and resentful, at a time when strong family unity is paramount.

I am thankful for the courage and strength of our family unit, which has always prevailed.

13
The Traveller

Catharine has always been cautious on steps and stairways and nervous of lifts, but she took her first aeroplane flight, at age seventeen, quite confidently.

John and Janine felt that it was time Noel and I had another break, and they assured us that Catharine would be quite safe to fly to Sydney. 'We'll be there to collect her as soon as the plane lands!' they promised.

With a little apprehension, we agreed, and proceeded to make the necessary arrangements. The service from Young was a small six-seater plane. The local booking agent, who was well known to us, reassured us that the pilot would indeed deliver Catharine from the plane to the pick-up area, into the safe hands of her brother. We secured a booking and prepared Catharine as best we could without wanting to alarm her.

On the appointed morning, we arrived at the airport early. There were two other passengers also waiting, who offered to keep an eye on Catharine during the flight. Noel spoke to the pilot, who agreed to deliver her to John. With a medal of Our Lady pinned to her collar, and many prayers, we waved her off.

A week later, we were at the airport to welcome the beaming young traveller home.

This was repeated two years later with confidence that all would be just a matter of routine. However, unbeknown to us, this time there was no stopover at Cowra, as there had been the last time, so the plane arrived in Sydney ahead of schedule. John and his boys had come a few minutes early to see the plane come in. As they made their way to the viewing window, John heard a familiar voice call his name. Glancing around, he spotted Catharine, waving and smiling from behind the attendant's desk, where the pilot had placed her for safe keeping until her brother arrived.

We became involved with Faith and Light, an international association of Christian communities for intellectually disabled people, their family and friends. They meet on a regular basis to celebrate the gift of one another. Faith and Light was founded in 1971 at Lourdes in France by a French-Canadian man called Jean Vanier. It came to Australia in 1978 and Young formed a community in 1993.

Through our involvement with Faith and Light, we travelled by road and rail to Canberra, Sydney, Broken Hill and Albury.

April 2001 saw Catharine and me jetting off to London en route to France as members of a thirty-four-strong Australian Faith and Light group. We travelled to take part in the Faith and Light international thirtieth anniversary Easter pilgrimage at Lourdes.

This was a wonderful experience, and something I would never have contemplated were it not for the strong sense of security which prevails within the Faith and Light 'family', wherever we are.

Catharine has travelled alone on buses to and from Canberra many times now. There always seems to be someone looking out for her. I pray daily to God to keep her safe. I truly believe He does, otherwise I could not let her out of my sight.

14
Special Occasions and Achievements

Catharine has always loved music and dance, performing in front of television's *Young Talent Time* program from an early age. At ten years of age, she took ballet lessons under the guidance of a special young lady, Lenore McGlynn. One afternoon, I took Catherine along just to watch the girls. It wasn't long before she was behind the class following the children's steps. With the encouragement of Margurette McGlynn, the teacher's mother, who came to each class, we began to attend weekly lessons.

Catherine was bigger than the other girls in the class but wasn't bothered by that. She quickly picked up the routines. For the first three years, she did classical ballet, and then transferred to jazz ballet, which she preferred. Each year at the annual concert, Catherine was thrilled to perform on stage with her class. As she had attended many school concerts to witness her brothers and sister on stage at the town hall, it was very special for her to do the same.

Eventually, Lenore left Young, and Catherine attended old-time dances on a regular basis with her dad and me – she was content not to go on with the new ballet teacher. A few years later, she asked if she could try tap dancing. We approached the teacher, Mrs Pinda, who agreed to give her a try out with the ladies' class. However, knowing she wouldn't be able to achieve at that level, I intimated that it would be better for Catharine to start with a younger class. The girls accepted her, without question.

She learned tap for three years until Mrs Pinda transferred, and lessons ceased. As before, she was included in concerts. We then tried line dancing, but Catharine has a problem knee and the twisting caused it to ache, so we gave it up, even though we both enjoyed the dance and the company of the ladies who attended weekly with us.

For a few years, Catharine attended the Young School of Music. The first year, she tried singing. She loved to sing, but didn't know how to use her 'singing voice' as she calls it. She then went on to playing the recorder – again, a challenge she took on wholeheartedly and mastered.

In the Year of the Disabled, Catharine was invited to join the Girl Guides Association. She really enjoyed this experience. Generally she was well accepted by the girls, but three of them were especially kind and helpful to her. They were Sandra Bourke, Jacqueline Fathers and Sue Robinson (many thanks, girls). Attired in the Girl Guide uniform, Catharine attended weekly. She went on one weekend bivouac and enjoyed quite a few campfires and other Guiding pursuits. Catharine still speaks proudly of how she marched with the Guides each year in the Anzac Day march, 'Like Dad did.'

During her few years with the Guides, she was awarded four achievement badges – one for soft-toy making, one for craft and one for horse care, as well as a basic swimming skills badge. I do not wish to imply that any of this was easy; in fact, it was quite arduous and time-consuming for Catharine as well as for her teachers and me, but she was keen, so we persevered. As with all things she had learned, except TAFE, I had to attend all classes, observe and take notes. Not that I could do ballet or tap dancing, read music or play netball – but I could guide her in practice if I had some basic idea of the procedures. This meant that Noel was often left alone, but he understood and encouraged us all the way.

In 1985, Catharine attended a debutante ball with me to assist with the catering. As we watched the presentation of the debutantes, she made the now familiar comment, 'I could do that.' Here we go again, I thought, and accepted another challenge. Knowing she could 'do that', I turned it over in my mind before discussing it with her dad. He was all for the idea.

With the decision made and time on our side, the first step was to find a suitable dress. I chose not to attempt to make it myself, as it had to be special.

So, on our next visit to our son Peter and his new wife, De'hanne, in Sydney, I announced to Noel, 'We have to go into the city and buy Catharine a deb frock.'

I am not a city person – in fact, city crowds terrify me – but Noel was quite comfortable there. We set off with a list of possible shops to try, suggested by De'hanne. Hours – and many frocks – later, I was beginning to feel disheartened. Noel and Catharine were quite weary, the shop assistants tried their best – a tuck here, a frill there, but nothing suitable was to be found. There was one I considered; it was not white, but a deep cream.

'Let's take a breather and have some lunch while you give it some thought!' Noel suggested.

Refreshed from the short break, we soldiered on. There was one more shop on our list – Sugar House. Maryann's wedding frock and the one I wore to her wedding came from there ten years earlier. In we trooped. Again, racks and racks of frills, flounces, puffed sleeves and gathered skirts, again they did not look right.

'Perhaps this "special dress" doesn't exist,' I mused unhappily. I wandered around, examining every area in the shop, until I spotted a taffeta strapless frock, size 12 with a short-sleeved jacket. 'What about this one?' I questioned the sales lady, who by now was quite jaded by my rejection of all her best effects.

'Oh, that isn't really a deb frock,' she assured me.

'Let's try it on!' I suggested.

As Catharine is so short, the lady had her stand on a stool so that we could get a better idea without the skirts being crumpled. Out of the fitting room came Catharine and up onto the stool.

'This is it!' I exclaimed. 'It's just right!'

The fit and style were perfect, and all that was needed was five inches off the length, and tiny shoulder straps. I wasn't interested in the price – we had to have this one. With the purchase in a bag, we wearily made our way back to Riverwood before returning to Young the next day.

Shoes and gloves were purchased later, and again the search was on. As Catharine's shoe size was only one and a half, I did not expect there would be a great choice locally but, lo and behold, one local shop had just received a new line of white, low-heeled court shoes, the latest thing for teenagers, and, yes, they had the correct size. Perfect. The gloves were quite a different story. A friend in Sydney purchased the smallest ladies' elbow-length white gloves she could find, and sent them to us. The arm size was just right, but this young debutante-to-be had very short fingers. I proceeded to remake each finger to fit, with great results.

The day before the ball was Catharine's twentieth birthday. Maryann had arranged with her brothers to buy a string of pearls and earrings. They were the ideal finishing touch.

Vincent was to partner Catharine on the night of the Catholic Debutante Ball on 20th May 1986. He lived in Sydney and could not attend deb practice, so, in the weeks leading up to the ball, I filled in as her partner. The presentation Pride of Erin waltz was no problem, as Catharine was quite accomplished in all old-time dancing by then. She quickly picked up the entrance routine, and from her ballet days she already knew how to curtsy, so really it all ran smoothly. Vincent attended the final rehearsal the evening before the ball. All was in order.

The day dawned wet and gloomy. Catharine had a miserable head cold, but nothing daunted us. There had already been a trial run with the hairdresser, so, with the style selected, Anne was determined to do a special job on this customer. Catharine's hair was swept up in a circle of curls, and dotted with white flowers. The result was very becoming.

As we had a table reserved for sister, brothers, aunts and uncles, Noel and Vincent went a little earlier to get set up. Catharine and I were to take a taxi. Mr Mundy had been driving Catharine to and from school for many years, and therefore we engaged him for this important time. On arrival at the Town Hall, we were assembled upstairs for group photos. Nine o'clock eventually came around. I joined Noel and our guests and awaited the arrival of the official party, to be followed by the debutantes and partners. Being the shortest deb, Catharine was to be the first one presented. The master of ceremonies, Bill Kearney, took his place and introduced the official party. The flower girls (our granddaughter, Bridget, was one) and pageboys were in place. The pianist began to play the entrance music.

At last, there in the archway, stood Vincent and Catharine.

She still tells of the time, 'I wasn't nervous, but Vincent was.' A fact he readily agrees to.

Stepping onto the carpet, they proceeded slowly up the hall.

'The first debutante of the evening is Miss Catharine Keir, partnered by Mr Vincent Keir,' announced the MC, loud and clear.

Catharine wasn't expecting this. Her face lit up with a big smile, but she didn't miss a beat. As they reached the appointed spot, Vincent stepped aside, and Catharine moved forward and executed a graceful curtsy. The matron of honour, Wendy Hardy, came forward, took Catharine by the hand as had been rehearsed, and presented her to Father Kevin Flynn, who spoke a few words. Slowly, she moved back to take Vincent's arm, and they advanced to their specific place to stand while the other twenty-nine girls went through their paces. Then came the Pride of Erin – first with partners, then with the proud dads.

This was a magical night for Catharine and for us, with many congratulatory comments from those present. Vincent was surprised when some of his friends implied that it was good of him to partner her. He told them, 'I was proud to partner her!'

The photos of all the debutantes duly appeared in the local press. Many friends and acquaintances learned of Catharine's big night and offered their congratulations, and expressed pleasure that she was able to join with other young ladies in this step into social life.

Catharine attended many balls with Noel and me during the ensuing years. There were more lovely ball gowns, but the deb frock was often worn, until Catharine outgrew it.

I have gained much pleasure in choosing Catharine's clothes. My father advised me when she was young, 'Always dress her nicely – lots of families don't, you know.'

Dad need not have been concerned. Catharine's appearance has always been a family priority. My sisters have handed on the best of their daughter's clothes over the years. Most of her teenage wardrobe was from her well dressed cousins.

Catharine's 21st Birthday

Nineteenth May 1987 was the date of Catharine's twenty-first birthday. Previous family members' twenty-firsts had been celebrated at home, but this time I didn't feel able to manage. Here was this beautiful young woman who had emerged from the tiny, frail, black baby twenty-one years earlier – akin to a magnificent butterfly from its lowly origin. We decided to hold this important event at the Services and Citizens Club of which the three of us were members. A function room and menu were chosen, and a firm booking made.

The guest list was carefully selected. There were many people who had played roles in Catharine's development whom we wished to include. Her numerous relatives – Grandma, aunts, uncles, cousins, brothers, sister, nieces, nephews and their partners – had all taken an interest in this special girl from the very beginning. They all wished to join in this celebration with her.

Then, a frock befitting the occasion was needed. A few months earlier in the year, we were to attend the wedding of our godson, Tim, in Adelaide. This would be an opportune time to look in the shops as we travelled leisurely homewards.

As we gathered the evening before the wedding, the subject of Catharine's birthday came up. I mentioned that we were taking the opportunity of this trip to buy a frock.

'Catharine, we haven't seen your deb frock. I heard it was beautiful. Why not wear it for us?' suggested Auntie Mary Helen.

We considered this idea over the next few days and, as Catharine was keen at the prospect, we settled on this.

A friend, Paul Hewson, who is very talented with flowers, offered to do the floral arrangements in the Flamingo Room, where the party was to be held. Maryann baked and decorated the cake. We engaged Jim Anderson, who played the best old-time dance music in the area; we had danced to his band for years. Jim played piano for most deb ball presentations, and many weddings including Maryann's.

As 19th fell on Saturday, we chose to attend the 6 p.m. Vigil Mass before proceeding to the club. We were dressed in our party attire. Catharine attracted much attention and admiration, and revelled in informing everyone that we were going to 'the Club' for her twenty-first birthday party.

Before entering the room, Peter and De'hanne handed Catharine a posy to carry, and Uncle Peter Herbert, who had driven from Sydney to attend, pinned a lovely brooch on her shoulder. She was positively beaming as she greeted her guests.

That evening, as had her debut ball, proved to be a very special event. After the meal had been served and eaten, the official part of the evening came, where Catharine was toasted with moselle, the wine of her choice. The customary orations were given, and the cake cut. Catharine responded with a few well chosen words of her own before opening her gifts. We then took to the floor and danced the night away.

The gifts she received consisted of an assortment of jewellery. Anticipating this, Maryann had organised her brothers to join with her to purchase a beautiful, large, upright wooden jewellery case. The next day she assisted Catharine with setting out the many pieces in it.

Nine years later, with Catharine's thirtieth birthday nearing, family and friends were eager for a celebration, but Catharine announced, 'I don't want a party. I'd like to sleep on a ship like you and Dad did.' (We had taken a short cruise around Fiji some years earlier.)

Noel joked with her, 'That's easy! The next time you're in Sydney, we'll take a ferry ride and you can take your pillow!'

'Dad!' she protested. 'Not *that* kind of ship!'

We explored the possibilities and considered our options. An ocean cruise was more expensive than we could comfortably afford. A Hawkesbury river cruise seemed to be the answer. We enquired at the travel agent and learned that this service had been discontinued. So, with our best efforts thwarted, we proceeded to encourage the party idea.

Two weeks later, Noel was scanning the travel section of the Sunday paper and an article advertising a weekend cruise out of Sydney caught his attention. The date was after the birthday, but it seemed ideal and the price was right.

Hurriedly, we made the necessary arrangements and secured a booking for a four-berth cabin. We reasoned that if we took our eleven-year-old granddaughter, Keren, both she and Catharine could join in the activities, making things easier for Noel and me, and more enjoyable for Catharine.

The evening of the birthday, a few family members gathered for dinner. The main topic of conversation was the cruise in three months. The time passed swiftly, and soon we were packing and on our way to John's place. He was to deliver us to the ship in time to settle into our cabin. We entered through the terminal and so did not see much of the ship. Around seven-thirty that night, the vessel pulled away from its moorings. The lights around the Harbour, the Bridge and the Opera House were breathtaking. Our girls revelled in the excitement, as slowly the ship circled the Harbour and headed out to sea through the heads.

The first evening was spent exploring the ship, the *Karelia*, from stem to stern. This was a large cruise ship, so there was much to see. Seasickness became a problem for Keren and Noel as the weather became turbulent, so the ship's doctor had to be consulted. They could not tolerate the smell of hot food in the dining room. However, we did enjoy a poolside smorgasbord lunch on Saturday.

The wind had risen and whipped up the sea. Our glasses were frosted over with the salty spray, but we enjoyed the cruise. Our girls played deck games, as well as participating in line dancing, horse racing (shipboard style) and bingo, at which Catharine won thirty dollars. We took in a film in the picture theatre.

One look at the flashing lights of the casino and the colourful gaming tables convinced us it was not our scene. On the final evening, we were treated to a night club performance with top-class artists, which topped off an action-packed weekend.

Docking early Monday morning, we disembarked at 8. As we walked away, we were able to look back at the ship, and the girls were astonished at its size.

We returned home tired but very satisfied, and Catharine had thoroughly enjoyed her 'sleep on a ship', as did Keren. Noel and I had gained pleasure in indulging our girls and fulfilling a birthday wish!

15
Looking to the Future

The greatest concern, I dare to suggest, to all parents of disabled (especially intellectually disabled) offspring, is how to ensure that the care of those loved ones is continued should they outlive us. Noel and I always prayed for divine assistance in regard to our parenthood. As time passed, Catharine's well-being was paramount. There was no precedent we were happy with. It was some years before we discovered what we felt was an acceptable option.

From the time Catharine began school at Bellhaven, we became involved in meetings and committees regarding disabled people. Noel held the position of president of the Bellhaven committee for a number of years. He and I had attended national conferences in Sydney as delegates representing Young. We were also present at the first two Down Syndrome Association seminars held over weekends at the university in Sydney. These were great occasions for us, as we met many families with Down syndrome sons and daughters. We were amazed at the number of families – some childless but some with children of their own – who had adopted Down children. We realised how blessed we were, as Catharine had developed more skills than most others present.

About the time Catharine was thirteen years old, we heard of Mater Dei at Camden. Thinking it was for long-term residents, Noel rang and spoke to the superior, a Sister Paula, who explained that Mater Dei was a boarding school. She asked if we had heard of L'Arche.

'No. What can you tell me about it?' Noel responded.

'L'Arche are Christian-based. They have houses where carers and adults with an intellectual disability live in the community. There's a house in Canberra. Perhaps you might like to contact them. I could give you the phone number,' she offered.

'Thank you, I'd appreciate that,' Noel replied.

He hung up the phone and, before dialling the L'Arche number, told me what he had learned. The call was answered by Eileen Glass, who explained to him that she was the L'Arche coordinator, as well as a live-in assistant at their house in Gledden Street, Chifley, in Canberra. She was extremely gracious and suggested, 'Call, if ever you come to Canberra.'

Maryann lived in Canberra and we often visited her, so, on our next trip, Noel called L'Arche, to follow up the invitation. When he asked what day and time would be suitable for us to call, Eileen assured us, 'Just any time you want.'

I will always remember the warm-hearted welcome we received, and how quickly Catharine made herself at home. This was a five-bedroom house; there were three intellectually disabled adults in residence. Their policy was to take the most needy cases, and of course there was a waiting list.

By 12.30, we began preparing to leave, but Eileen insisted, 'No, you must join us for lunch.'

We protested, as we did not wish to be any bother.

'No bother at all. We all make our own lunch here,' we were told.

With this agreed, we were soon seated around the large wooden table laid with bread, butter, cheese and salad. Eileen went to fetch Kaleen, who was not well and had spent the morning in bed.

'It's good for her to join us,' she explained.

After grace was said, we set about making our own sandwiches. Kaleen, also a Down syndrome young lady, sat at the end of the table. Eileen, sitting next to her, quietly asked what she would like on her sandwich. We were impressed with this lady's gentle manner as she coaxed and guided Kaleen to prepare and eat her own lunch.

The love and care experienced in that house made a deep and lasting impression on Noel and me. As we drove away, we agreed that this is what we had been searching for. Unfortunately, Catharine's chances of ever living there were very slim indeed, but we did write to the director and have her name recorded on the waiting list.

As time passed, we enquired why there were not more L'Arche homes opening up. We were told that Jean Vanier, the founder, had a wonderful spirituality and had clear visions that these homes would have a real community spirit, where assistants live and share their lives with the disabled. This life does not appeal to many, and staffing is carefully chosen and monitored. We asked if it would be possible to have a L'Arche home at Young. We were informed that the policy is that, before any consideration could be given, the proposed live-in coordinator of a new community must spend two years living and working in an established community. Could we find such a person?

With this in mind, Noel arranged an evening at the Bellhaven School with Eileen Glass as guest speaker. Before becoming interested in L'Arche, Eileen was a successful high school teacher. During a holiday overseas, she spent some time in a L'Arche community. Like Jean Vanier before her, she was drawn to this special way of life, of people giving generously of their extraordinary talents and time to enrich the lives of intellectually disabled people, who many others give little thought or care toward.

As the result of the Bellhaven meeting, a steering committee was formed to investigate the possibility of setting up a privately run L'Arche-type home at Young. After many months, meetings, phone calls and letters, the Housing Commission agreed to supply a purpose-built house for our needs. We set about drawing up a suitable, no-frills plan, which was submitted. After some time, we were informed by the commission that they would draw up their own plan and have their architect meet with us. To our committee, the department's design was unnecessarily elaborate, but we could not convince them to modify it. Eventually the house was built, and government funding for furnishing and one staff was forthcoming.

In the interim, we were offered an existing four-bedroom house to begin our enterprise. This was an exciting time for parents in Young. We envisioned that our young adults would be able to stay near home while making their new homes in a fully supervised, family-type atmosphere. Our temporary dwelling, 'Bellhaven Cottage', was furnished, and a local lady,

Maureen Cummins, was employed on a five-day, 3 p.m. to 9 a.m. basis, as the residents went to work daily. We opened with Francis and Mathew in residence and one room for respite care.

This venture received great support, our carer proved to be first rate, and the house was just as welcoming and homely as we had hoped. A year later, Dianne joined the household. Maureen, and later Helen Curtis, assisted her to adapt and she settled in. In due course, our new house was completed and our people moved on.

A plan to offer full-time accommodation was begun, funding for a part-time staff member was acquired and plans were ongoing for another full-time carer and further residents. At about this juncture, a rift occurred in the committee and, much to our distress, our special project home was signed over to the Lambing Flat Enterprise, who conducted the sheltered workshop and assisted accommodation in Young. They agreed that there was a need for a full-time care facility, which fitted their charter.

Noel and I were deeply grieved by this turn of events but, as it was still to operate along the same lines, with Helen retained on staff, all had not been lost.

It was not many months before full-time care was withdrawn and all of our good work undone. Lambing Flat Enterprises relinquished their lease on the building in early 2001. The building is now Carers Lodge and is run by the Young Community Carers Group Inc. with the support of the Mental Health Department.

The next avenue we explored was for a religious-owned and run full-time care facility. I mentioned it to the combined church women's group and spoke to a Catholic Women's League Conference about the urgent need to find safe accommodation for these special people whom God has placed in our care. The conference passed a motion to approach our Catholic bishop to explore possible avenues. Presently, Sister Jeanie Heininger, a nun of the Good Samaritan order, was employed to assess the needs of people with disabilities in this archdiocese.

Soon after this, we were invited to set up a meeting at Young. We contacted ten families who we knew were as interested as we were. Sister Jeanie arrived and spent a few hours with us. She met with us almost monthly over a period of eighteen months, to ascertain the need in country areas for full-time Christian-based care. We were then advised how to approach our local parish councils. Sister Jeanie had great knowledge and affinity with intellectually disabled people, and offered us much support and encouragement. During one of her visits, she mentioned that she had been the principal of the Camden Mater Dei School. Noel told her he had spoken to Sister Paula a few years earlier.

'Really!' she laughed. 'That was me. I've gone back to my family name but I was Sister Paula then.'

Through her work, some assisted-care homes have opened in the ACT, but Young is still without supervised accommodation that we consider suitable for our daughter. At first, our parish committee were very keen to support the idea but, as time passed and members changed, the interest waned and was forgotten. Unfortunately, the Catholic schools eat up most of the finances in country towns, making it difficult to have projects like this one considered.

During Sister Jeanie's visits, she asked if we were aware of Faith and Light. 'It's a worldwide body founded by Jean Vanier, the founder of L'Arche.'

'No, we haven't heard of Faith and Light, but we know about L'Arche.'

Sister explained that Faith and Light is where people with intellectual disability, their family and friends come together and celebrate the gift of one another, with shared prayer, friendship and a meal. Faith and Light has a specific charter. The idea is to organise a monthly gathering comprised of one-third parents, one-third disabled and one third friends.

Under Sister Jeanie's guidance, we began a Faith and Light community in 1995, and it is still in operation as I write. In the first year, we joined the Canberra L'Arche group for a weekend at the Galong Monastery. This proved to be a great success, and our affinity with the ACT is ongoing.

During the Galong weekend, Catharine took a fancy to a lady who was a carer with the Canberra group. Catharine invited her to come and visit one day. I was informed of this, and in subsequent conversation determined that Catharine's new friend was Angela Capes, a New Zealander. She was living at the Chifley Street L'Arche house with the intention of setting up a community in New Zealand. She was very happy to visit Catharine on her next two-day break and did so, staying in her flat.

Consequently, she invited Catharine to visit Chifley Street as her guest when she could arrange a bed. This occurred a few weeks later. Our link with L'Arche was renewed. By then, there were three houses in Canberra. Angela visited Catharine again before returning to New Zealand, where she has now established a L'Arche home.

Early one morning, a few months later, we received a phone call from Sister Jeanie.

'The coordinator of L'Arche has just asked me if I know of a girl with some self-care skills who might be interested in making her home at L'Arche. I immediately thought of Catharine, and your thoughts on the L'Arche concept.'

'I don't think we're ready,' was my surprised answer.

Laughingly, she offered, 'Will you ever be?'

To which I had to admit, 'I don't suppose we will, but we have to give this some thought.'

As we considered the idea, Noel and I both came to realise that now was the optimum time in what would be a very big step in Catharine's life. When the call came from the coordinator of L'Arche a few hours later, we had made our decision and accepted her invitation to give Catharine the opportunity offered.

'This necessitates a long, gentle process,' she told us. 'Let's begin by having Catharine come for weekend visits now and then, and see how she fits in.'

The occasional visits became monthly, and Catharine was really enjoying her time there. At Easter 1996, we joined in a national pilgrimage at Broken Hill to celebrate twenty-five years of Faith and Light. The L'Arche communities were there also, and Catharine spent all the time she could in their company. All was going well, and we could imagine that soon

Catharine would spend more and more time at L'Arche. However, she had been experiencing mysterious pain for some months, and her doctor could not pinpoint the cause. The attacks became more frequent and severe, and she was not able to visit as often as before. Eventually, just when she was due for a six-week stay at L'Arche, her doctor diagnosed gallstones, and placed her on the waiting list for surgery.

Unfortunately for us, there was another girl whose family was keen to have her join L'Arche, and Catharine lost out on the placing. We still kept in touch and, when she had recovered from her illness, she visited now and then. As always, we prayed that Catharine would have the opportunity to live in a full-time care facility like L'Arche before the time came when we were unable to care for her properly ourselves. I was feeling the strain of keeping up the support necessary to allow her to live the life she was used to, but we carried on as usual.

Noel had taken up a hobby in recycled woodwork, in which he was skilled. I was enjoying my needlework and quilt making. Catharine, with the five gallstones removed and on display in a jar, enjoyed life to the full.

16
That Special Holiday

The summer of 1997–1998 was extremely hot and dry. Noel had been suffering with prostate problems for some months and was seeing a urologist with a view to surgery soon. He was very productive in his workshop, creating some lovely items – mirrors, blanket boxes, coat stands and frames for Catharine's long-stitch pictures among them. Between this, playing bowls three times a week and tennis twice weekly, he was very fit.

Our seventeenth grandchild was to be baptised on the first weekend in February at Lake Macquarie, where Vincent and his family lived. The hot weather was still with us and we really were not keen to pack our bags and set out just then. Our grandchildren are very special to us, though, and we had not missed a baptism for any trivial reason yet, and we were not about to let the heat stop us.

How to travel, we wondered – by train or car? Our decision to take the trip in our one-ton ute was made, because there were a few things Noel wanted to get to people along the way. The evening before we were to leave home, we loaded up the ute with a deep freeze refrigerator, a large square chicken coop complete with a hen and two chickens, a large blanket box and a box of tools, plus our cases.

Our neighbour, Stephen, who had come to collect a house key so he could attend to Tommy, Catharine's dog, laughed when he saw the load, saying, 'All you need is Edna in the rocking chair on the top and you could be the Beverley Hillbillies.'

The next morning, equipped with a large container of iced water and a box of sandwiches, we set out. As the vehicle only had a fan and no air-conditioning, we were pleased there was a little cloud cover overhead.

Arriving in Goulburn at midday, and following pre-acquired instructions, we found the home of Tony Keir, Noel's second cousin, where we were to deliver the blanket box. Noel had constructed it from timber recycled from an old house on the property of Tony's parents and grandparents before them. The box was unloaded, admired and gratefully received by Tony and his wife. By now it was lunchtime, so we took our sandwiches and shared a pleasant hour with the other Keir family before setting out again.

Our next stop was Cobbitty, where Peter and his family had their home – this was where the hen and chickens were destined. We promptly unloaded them in readiness to surprise the boys who were due home from school shortly. Peter, De'hanne and sons Ambrose and Rhyse had recently built and taken up residence on a small acreage. The boys had a horse each, and some chickens definitely added to the farm atmosphere.

Over the next few days of our stay, Peter and his dad spent much of their time outdoors, discussing horse care, the chicken pen, tree planting and general land care. Noel and I agreed that we had not seen Peter so relaxed for a long time. Rural living was to his liking, having grown up on the land. His family also enjoyed this lifestyle, and have all become accomplished horse riders.

The baptism was to be on Sunday. We drove to Riverwood to spend Saturday night with John, Janine and sons, Luke, Shane and Joel. Rising early Sunday, we set off for Newcastle. On reaching the church, we were met by Peter and family, who had travelled up, as well as my brother Ron and members of his family, who lived nearby, and joined by friends of Sue and Vincent.

Following the ceremony, we all returned to the house, where a very pleasant family day was enjoyed. Before leaving for their respective homes, the boys unloaded the last of our cargo – the deep freezer – which was for Vincent and Sue.

Noel, Catharine and I stayed on for a week, during which time Noel and Vincent put together an older-style garden shed which Ron had given them. They also did some necessary work on the roof of the house. Noel was very happy, as he was not one to sit around, and Vincent much appreciated his dad's time, acquired knowledge and skill. During our stay, we spent time with Ron and his wife, Shirley, relaxing in pleasant conversation, savouring the opportunity just to be together.

Contrary to my usual policy, I took quite a few photos – Noel was much the better photographer but, on this trip, I seemed to be the one with the camera in hand.

Vincent and Sue's home is a well set-out family home with overhead fans in the bedrooms, so, even though the hot weather persisted and the humidity was high, the cooler evenings and fans afforded restful sleep, which by the end of our stay had rejuvenated us.

On our return journey, as always on starting out on a trip, we prayed, asking Our Lady for protection as we travelled. Noel was keen to show Catharine Wiseman's Ferry. Following directions from Vincent, we set off. As we approached the bridge at Swansea, we had to stop, as it was opening up to allow a boat to pass through. Overhead, on the tall light standards either side of us, sat large pelicans.

'Watch out, Catharine. Close the window,' Dad said. 'Look up there. I hope they don't drop a big mess on us.'

'Dad!' She was shocked. 'Don't be silly.'

'Well, they might!' he teased.

We watched the boat appear again, and the bridge slowly returned back in place. We moved on, travelling the Pacific Highway until we found ourselves at Wyong, where we stopped for a drink.

Noel enquired for further directions to Wiseman's Ferry, realising that this was not the way Vincent had suggested. Somehow, we had taken the wrong highway. Nevertheless, we had plenty of time, and we were enjoying the scenery. Again we veered off-course and found ourselves travelling through a beautiful lush area with lovely horses and cattle. We witnessed turf being harvested on two different properties.

Had we been in our car as we usually were, Catharine would not have seen any of this – she would have been asleep on the back seat. She did not enjoy travelling but, from her vantage spot between Noel and me, she was enjoying the trip, and a lively banter continued between us.

Some of the road we encountered was gravel. Even though we realised we were off the direct road, Noel knew we were headed in the right direction.

'Are we lost?' queried Catharine at one stage.

'No, not lost – just on the wrong road,' her dad reassured her.

I had no worries, with full confidence that Noel knew where he was. The road was slow and extremely winding. We arrived at the ferry at midday. It was just unloading at the opposite bank, then we watched it edging slowly towards us, carrying a few vehicles. Noel explained to Catharine that we were going across to the other side on it.

'How?' she puzzled.

'Just wait and see,' he advised.

There were a few cars ahead of us, so she could not really see the docking area until it was our turn to go on board. We took our place in the centre. Nothing seemed to be happening. As we drew away from the dock, we got out and stood at the rail.

When Catharine realised we were moving and surrounded by water, she exclaimed, 'I can't believe it, I just can't believe it.'

We had only taken a few photos when it was time to prepare to drive off and up the other side. The climb off the ferry and up into the street was steep. We were hot, thirsty and hungry – our next pressing need was some refreshment. The only food sign was on a very steep grade, so Noel drove on, only to find we were soon out of the village area. There was no alternative but to retrace our track. We found a parking spot under a small tree not far from the shop where we were able to buy a sandwich and cold drink.

Back on the road, our intention was to drive to Jenolan Caves. Noel had been talking about taking Catharine to see the caves for two years, but we had not done so. He had decided that now was the opportune time. As we neared Penrith, Noel suggested we should find a motel, as he was feeling tired. To our amazement, the odd motels we did see displayed No Vacancy signs. We pulled into a tourist information centre to be informed that there probably would not be a vacant room between Penrith and Bathurst, as it was St Valentine's Day. Noel worried where we would find a place to stay, saying he was getting weary and could sleep on the truck, but not Catharine and me.

As we got back on the road, I began to pray, 'Please God, find us a room – any room.'

Driving through Springwood, I spotted a Vacancy sign in front of a motel. Gratefully, we pulled into the yard to find there was one family suite available. We took the key and unloaded our bags, then showered and refreshed ourselves. Noel lay on the bed as I turned the television on. The reception was bad on the only one channel we could get. The small refrigerator was frosted up. I put some water in, so that we could soon have a cold drink. This proved to be a vain hope, as even the next morning it was not much colder.

The motel restaurant was very up-market. Not feeling like dressing up, we ventured down the road a little to the only other shops – a service station and a small takeaway food outlet. We returned to our room with a barbecued chicken, a loaf of bread, some margarine and a jar of jam, which provided our dinner and breakfast as well.

To the delight of Catharine, the TV channel had *Xena*, a program Noel and I had not watched but she enjoyed. Needless to say, we endured it this once, Noel falling asleep halfway through.

Always the early riser, Noel had us on the move in good time next morning – hoping to find a church along the way where we could attend Mass. As we continued our journey, I glanced through a booklet depicting the area, noting the signposts. One little town ran into the next.

'Didn't Catharine come here somewhere for a holiday with LFE?' asked Noel.

'That's right,' I recalled.

'You came with Robin and Dianne. Do you remember?'

'Yes!' Catharine responded. 'It was at Lawson.'

Quickly, I consulted the brochure to discover that we were very near there.

All the while on the lookout for a Catholic church, we noticed quite a few cars parked on either side of the road up ahead.

'This might be one,' I speculated.

As we slowly drove past the sign, we read 'Santa Maria'.

'That's the name of the place where you stayed, Catharine. There must be Mass on now,' I suggested.

Noel drove down a lane and around behind the larger building, which was the Good Samaritan Sisters Convent. Parking the truck, we made our way through the yard to the front door of the church. Mass had just begun. People stood in the porch as we squeezed inside. Noel spotted a seat toward the front and indicated I take it. He and Catharine stayed at the back. As people moved forward for Holy Communion, I noticed Sister Joanne, a Good Samaritan nun we had met several times at Young. She had been living at the Community House in Canberra and was a good friend and supporter of Faith and Light.

After Mass, we had not caught up with Sister Joanne, and Noel suggested we look for her. As we made tracks back toward our vehicle, again through the yard, Catharine began to recognise the surroundings and was anxious to show us around.

The largest building used to be a boarding facility for schoolgirls but now was a holiday centre for disadvantaged groups, hence the time Catharine spent there. In answer to our knock, a surprised Sister Joanne opened the door. Greeting us warmly, she insisted we come inside and have a cup of tea. Catharine was very much at home and keen to show us where she slept on her visit. We were given a full tour of the complex and an invitation to return for a relaxing holiday sometime soon.

There had been a small shed converted into a prayer room with a large glass area overlooking the mountainside. Noel picked up some timber, intending to make a large cross for the wall of this room on returning home. Before leaving, I took another photo – this time of Noel, Catharine and Sister Joanne.

Planning to be at Jenolan Caves by lunchtime, we took our leave. Anyone who has travelled the road to Jenolan Caves would know that it is extremely steep and winding, requiring concentration and a steady hand to negotiate.

Our intention was to spend the night. While not sure about the available accommodation, Noel drove through and up onto the public parking area, which is a long, steep walk from the buildings.

We walked down and secured a booking for one night's stay at Jenolan House. We bought tickets for the 2.30 p.m. cave tour and enjoyed lunch in the cafeteria. I was surprised at how hot and humid it was. Noel decided to move the truck to the designated parking area behind the accommodation. Catharine and I elected to wait in the shade. I was becoming quite anxious by the time he returned, as he was away much longer than I had expected. I thought he was only going behind the guesthouse.

'Where have you been?' I asked.

'It's a damn long drive and walk back, past a few buildings, a motel and backpack-type accommodation,' he explained. 'You should see all the flash motorbikes back there,' he told Catharine, who liked motorbikes. Vincent rode a bike for years, and she loved a pillion ride whenever possible.

After a short break, we strolled down under the arch and settled down on a bench to wait for our tour to begin. The caves all open onto this area, so there were a number of people waiting.

Catharine engaged in conversation with a lady. I think she came from Canada.

'Have you been here before?' the lady enquired.

'Mum and Dad have, but not me!' Catharine answered.

'Are you scared?' the lady asked.

'I am, yes, a bit,' Catharine admitted.

'Well, that's OK,' responded the lady. 'We can be scared together. That'll be all right.'

Suddenly there was a rumbling sound as the motorbikes came down the grade. They reached the underground section where we were and revved their engines, reared up on their back wheels and roared up and out the other side. The sound reverberating around the rocky amphitheatre was deafening for some moments.

Catharine enjoyed their display, but her new-found friend was shocked.

'Don't they know how dangerous that is? Back home they'd be charged for endangering the public. That could well set off a rockslide in a place like this,' she told us.

Just then, our tour was announced. We assembled at the entrance to be instructed by our guide on how to proceed and what to expect. Noel and I tried to stay close to the front to allow Catharine to hear what was being said, and gain as much as possible from the experience.

'Don't be afraid to ask questions as we go along,' advised our guide.

The deeper we went, the cooler it became.

Catharine took everything in and kept exclaiming, 'That's amazing!'

The tour took one hour, and often as we moved along, Catharine would query the guide on various questions that popped into her active imagination.

'You did offer!' I jested.

The guide smiled, assuring me, 'It's quite OK!'

It was very damp and slippery in some areas, with many steep, narrow steps in quite confined spaces which were dimly lit. We expected that Catharine would be apprehensive in such an unfamiliar place, but she was so interested in it all that the time passed quickly. We emerged all too soon. We decided to explore the area outside, as it was still early. There are many walking tracks with little rippling streams, fish and bird life. But the last two days had been long and hot, and Noel and I, feeling fatigued, finally decided to call it a day.

First, Noel made the long trek to retrieve something we needed from the truck. Catharine and I started off to accompany him and to see the other buildings, but light rain began to fall and Noel insisted, 'You girls go back and get under cover.'

On his return, we enjoyed a meal before retiring for an early night. There was no TV in our room, so, while Noel turned in, I took Catharine downstairs. We watched a little TV and played a game of pool before deciding to go to bed also.

In the morning, we packed up our belongings and deposited them in the office before setting off for one last climb up the mountainside. Only one of the double doors was open. As we walked out, Catharine stepped over the edge of the low ramp, falling heavily on the paving. Gathering her up, we helped her back inside and sat her down to ascertain her injuries. Her ankle had been twisted, her little toe hurt, and there were abrasions on her arm and hip.

'I'm sorry, Mum,' she whimpered, trying to put on a brave face.

'It's OK, darling,' I consoled, as Noel removed her shoe and sock. 'We don't have to go walking.'

'But I want to,' she replied.

There appeared to be no real damage done. Soon she felt ready for a short walk, even though she was limping slightly. I pointed out to Noel where the ramp was four or five inches narrower than the doorway. By taking the climb in short bursts and rests, we reached the summit. As we did so, Catharine began to feel faint and to vomit. We were quite concerned but reassured her that she would feel better in a minute. After a rest, she brightened up and enjoyed the beautiful view with us. Though steep, the descent was much easier than the climb, and we took it slowly.

We arrived back at the guest house with a pale, very lame girl. As we walked onto the paved area, we noticed that the ramp had been moved, leaving an obvious wide gap beside the unopened door. Noel felt he must make an official report in case there might have been a broken bone in her foot. Thankfully, this was not the case – just some discoloration and soreness for a few days.

Our journey homeward took us through Bathurst and Cowra – another tourist attraction we had not visited was the Japanese Gardens there. Although hot and weary, we could not pass them by. The nice part of the garden was the many fish, which would quickly appear when a few crumbs of specially provided food was sprinkled into the water. We arrived home on Monday afternoon, following a most pleasant, eventful two days.

This twelve-day holiday, though reluctantly taken, turned out to be very memorable – a special time for us all, one that I have come to treasure as I often go over it in my mind. In light of what followed, I know it was providential.

The trying weather continued, and we settled back into our familiar routine.

17
Our Great Loss

Three weeks after our return, Noel told me he thought he should consult his doctor.

'Why?' I asked in surprise.

He said he was just a bit concerned.

'Would you like me to go with you?' I asked.

'Yes, if you like.'

An appointment was made for later in the day.

As Doctor ushered us into his room, he asked, 'What's your problem, Noel?'

To which Noel answered, 'I'm having difficulty driving. On a recent trip, I found myself misjudging corners and curves and now, since coming home, it's still happening.'

I was amazed. We had been around a myriad of curves and corners and I had not noticed any irregularity in his driving. I said nothing.

The doctor tested his balance, ears and eyes. He also carried out various other tests. 'Noel, I can't detect any reason for your dilemma. Perhaps you have a mild case of Ménières. If so, it may right itself. If not, see me again in a couple of weeks, and we'll look further.'

We took our leave and I did not give it much more thought, accepting the doctor's advice.

As I mentioned earlier, Noel was in the process of preparing to have prostate surgery soon. In the interim, he found the condition worsened markedly, causing both of us to lose a lot of sleep. Two weeks after his visit to Doctor regarding his driving problem, he became very tired and listless.

'This damn prostate and the heat are taking it out of him!' I surmised, thankful that it would soon be attended to.

Even though he played bowls and tennis, and continued his woodwork as usual, by the weekend he spent most of his time in the house, not getting up to play tennis on Saturday morning. He watched football on Sunday afternoon and insisted we go for a walk to stretch his legs. We were both alarmed at how weak he had become over a short period.

Monday morning, after another sleepless night, Noel developed the shakes. His whole body trembled, just from the effort of getting dressed. I had taken Catharine to croquet and was shocked to find him in this condition on my return.

'Noel, you're ill!' I stated the obvious.

'Yes, you'd better take me to the doctor.'

Three-thirty in the afternoon was the earliest appointment we could get. Noel improved slightly during the day.

Doctor suggested I get him to Wagga for a head scan. 'You may have had a slight stroke,' he told him.

The next day, I took him to Wagga for the scan. On Wednesday we received the diagnosis. The scan had shown a brain tumour.

On Thursday, Michael had us in Sydney at 12.30 to consult a neurologist at St Vincent's Hospital. The news was all bad. Noel had to be admitted on Sunday for a biopsy on Monday morning. Stunned, we returned to our son John's home in Riverwood.

As soon as I had received the result of the scan on Wednesday, I contacted Michael, who came, and I rang my sister Mary, in Forbes.

I had contacted them both the previous evening to warn them of my fears. 'Mary, I need you to come and get Catharine for me. Noel has a brain tumour.'

'We'll come immediately!' promised Mary.

Catharine was at TAFE and had no idea of our bad news. Before I told her, I wanted to have time to come to grips with what we were facing. By the time Catharine had come from TAFE, her Auntie Mary, whom she loves, was there. I told her she could go and spend a few days with Auntie Mary while Dad and I had a trip to Sydney. She knew her dad was not well, but soon got caught up in the excitement of a holiday at Forbes.

Just before Mary, Ron and Catharine left, we had the appointment in Sydney confirmed. We were all in shock and automatically went through the necessary preparations, to leave early the next morning.

As we neared Goulburn on the trip to Sydney, Noel said, 'Catharine should have been told more!'

'I'll tell her as soon as I can!' I promised him. Sitting in the back, I was thinking, 'It isn't something I can just land on her without the time to help her through it.'

That evening, when we had all tried to compose ourselves and support each other, I took John aside and told him I needed some privacy to ring Catharine. He showed me into his office.

'I don't know what I can say to her, John. You pray while I speak to her!'

Mary answered the phone and I explained the situation, warning, 'I have to tell Catharine. She'll be very upset, so be prepared for a difficult time.'

'You aren't going to tell her anything she doesn't already suspect,' Mary assured me. 'We've been having long talks and she's well aware her dad's very sick. Here she is!'

'Hello, Mum,' came down the phone. 'How's Dad?'

'He's very sick, darling. He has to go into hospital, so we have to stay in Sydney for a while. How are you?'

'I'll be all right with Auntie Mary. She's just like you – she looks like you and she talks like you,' she reassured me. After a few minutes' conversation, she said, 'Goodbye, Mum. Give Dad my love!'

I silently thanked God. As I left the office, John was waiting.

'How did it go?' he asked.

'She's amazing. She was the one helping me.'

On Friday, the rest of our family assembled at John's. They were convinced Catharine should be with us. Michael was returning to Young and coming back on Sunday morning. I arranged for him to bring Catharine back with him. On the way, he told her what to expect, so she was quite prepared. After a few tears, she coped really well.

Noel was pleased to have his entire family, grandchildren as well, around him in those difficult days. We all attended Mass with him on Sunday morning and had lunch together, before taking him to Saint Vincent's Hospital.

After the biopsy result on Wednesday, which confirmed the worst possible news, Noel decided to go along with the suggestion that six weeks' radiation might halt the growth a little. 'If you think it might help, I'll give it a go.'

Our family then returned to their respective homes.

During the next eight weeks, Maryann, our sons and grandchildren visited every week, often staying overnight to see us again the next day. Catharine spent most of the time in Forbes with my sisters, Mary and Janet, but was able to get to Sydney twice more.

After travelling into the hospital by train daily for two weeks from Riverwood, I was offered accommodation in a flat belonging to the hospital. I stayed there for forty days. Catharine was able to spend one night with me there.

It was just eight weeks from when we went to Sydney to 18th May, when we returned via air ambulance and Noel was admitted to the Mercy Care Centre at Young, where he spent six weeks before passing away on 27th June. A few days after our return, my sisters brought Catharine home. We were able to have Noel home for a few hours some days.

Twenty-eighth May was our forty-ninth wedding anniversary, which Catharine made sure was celebrated. She cooked a special lunch, complete with a bottle of apple cider (our usual celebratory drink). She set the table with our best silver cutlery and wine glasses. Michael brought Noel from the hospital. I am not sure Noel realised what the occasion was, but we did our best to make it special.

Catharine proposed a toast, 'To Mum and Dad, for their wedding anniversary.'

We clinked our glasses, and I drank the toast with mixed feelings, knowing there was not going to be a fiftieth. But, at the same time, I felt grateful for the many years which we had been blessed to share.

During those six weeks, we spent many hours at the hospital. Catharine would bring her long-stitch or books, and made many cups of tea and coffee for me in the hospital tea room. Noel enjoyed having her near. As he grew weaker, he stopped speaking; but to our surprise, he often had words for Catharine. She would come to the hospital from TAFE or day care every day. On hearing her voice greeting the nurses in the passage, Noel would brighten up and acknowledge her as she appeared in the door.

Just a few days before he passed away, she greeted him saying, 'I love you, Dad!'

He responded quite clearly, 'I love you, too!' This was amazing, as he had not spoken for some days.

Even though Catharine was well aware of Dad's decline, and had her tearful times, she showed great strength and compassion.

The afternoon before he died, she said to him, 'You'll soon see your mum Constance, now, Dad,' and patted his hand.

Noel's mother had died when he was two years old. I do hope he heard her. He would have been so proud of her faith and understanding.

As we were ordering flowers for the funeral, Catharine asked that three special flowers be bought. 'For me, Mum and Maryann,' she explained.

We were not sure what her intentions were, but the flowers were ordered.

Later, while discussing who would take part in the Mass, she announced, 'Me, Maryann and Bridget will do the offertory.'

Again no one argued, pleased that she wished to take part.

Some family members did readings. All the grandchildren carried a flower in the offertory procession, which they placed in a basket near the altar. I had not thought to mention this to Catharine and instruct her of the procedure when so many would follow her. Until now, it had always just been Catharine, Noel and me at Sunday Mass.

Undaunted, she took her position and led the way to the altar, presented her offering to Father Peter My, who greeted and thanked her. This is when I thought she would be confused. But no, she moved to the extreme left to make room for the others, and waited as if she had rehearsed. When all were in line beside her, having deposited their flowers, Catharine reverently bowed. All followed her lead. She then returned to the seat beside me. She answered all the responses and sang all the hymns.

It was not until we were outside the church as we walked hand in hand following the coffin that she began to cry. At the hearse, she put her head in her hands on the coffin and sobbed.

Father Peter gently said, 'Give her time. She's all right.'

A few moments passed, she lifted her head and I held her until her sobs subsided. She indicated to Maryann and me to place our flowers on the coffin with hers.

The undertaker then offered Catharine a small bottle, saying, 'Would you like to sprinkle Dad's coffin with holy water, Catharine?'

'Yes, please!' was the tearful reply, and she did.

She still speaks about the holy water. It was a special moment for her. Soon she was engulfed in family and friends with hugs and kisses for us all. At the graveside, she conducted herself admirably. In fact, she endured the entire episode of Noel's illness and passing with remarkable faith and courage.

In the weeks following, there were many friends and family around us. Eventually, it was just Catharine and me. We shared our loss and comforted each other day by day. Then I noticed a change in her.

She became withdrawn, yet kept asking, 'Are you all right, Mum?'

She knows me so well – there is no hiding anything from her. On questioning whether she was all right, she reluctantly confided in me that someone had told her, 'You're an adult now – you must look after Mum, let her have some time to herself.'

I was shocked and at a loss to understand such insensitivity. I could only assume she has misunderstood the advice given to her by this person.

Catharine and I have a special bond even some members of the family do not comprehend. We are always open and honest with each other. I assured her that she must come to me at any time.

'We should talk about our feelings, and if we feel like crying, we should!'

From then on, that's what we did.

After such a session, she would dry her eyes and say, 'I feel better now, Mum.'

For a long time, upsetting dreams she had about people mistreating her Dad troubled Catharine. Then, one morning, she said, 'I had a nice dream about Dad. I dreamed that you and Dad were dancing at the Town Hall.'

We built on this by recalling the good times, and it seemed to help us both.

When Noel had realised and accepted his condition was indeed fatal, his concern was for me. 'I want you to buy yourself a new car,' he told me.

'The old one will do me – I won't drive far,' I protested.

'No, you'll want to go to Forbes. I don't want you on the road in the old car – it's worn out.'

He was adamant, so I agreed. To make certain, when we were all together at the hospital, he said to the family, 'Be sure and see that Mum gets a new car.'

Another day he said, 'I wish we had Catharine settled for you.'

'Don't worry, Noel. It will happen,' I tried to reassure him.

Soon after Noel's death, Michael and John arranged the purchase of the new car according to their father's wishes. I had just celebrated my seventieth birthday. Catharine insisted that the car was Dad's birthday present to me.

18
Life Goes On

Just six months had passed and we were getting on with our new lifestyle, when I received a phone call from the Canberra L'Arche community leader.

She was well aware of our situation. 'Do you still want Catharine to come to L'Arche?' she asked. 'We have a placement coming up soon.'

At first all I could think of was 'Not now, not yet,' but I knew that the reality was that this opportunity might not arise for years. Mindful of Noel's wishes, and painfully aware that my life could be taken just as suddenly as his had been, it was crystal clear what my response had to be.

'Well, yes!' I began. 'I'm not sure if this is a good time, though. I'll have to talk it over with Catharine. Can I get back to you?'

'Of course,' she replied. 'Take a little time. We would love to have her, you know.'

I pondered and prayed on how best to approach Catharine. At first, I did not mention full-time living – just suggested weekends, as before.

She was keen, remembering her previous visits. 'Will you be all right by yourself?' was her query, a concern she still has.

'I have lots of things to do to keep me busy,' I assured her.

The weekend stays began immediately. It was December 1998. By April 1999, we had moved her TV, Grandma's chair and some of her personal belongings. She was living full-time at the L'Arche community home in Chifley, ACT.

The first few months were happy, but as the novelty wore off she became homesick. She worried even more that I was lonely and needed her. Though this was quite true, I would tell her, 'Yes, I do miss you, and I miss your sister and brothers too. That's what happens when children grow up. You all need to have a home of your own, where you can get jobs. You know that's what Dad and I want for you. I am OK, really.'

'You are still my mum, aren't you?' she asked one day.

'I'll always be your mum, like I'm Maryann's and the boys' mum and they've been married a long time,' I tried to explain.

Still today there are numerous phone calls. 'Mum, I miss you.'

But with a routine of work and various activities to occupy her, she is coping better. There are many ups and downs. Maryann keeps in close contact with Catharine and me.

Each month, Catharine comes home by Countrylink coach or I drive down and stay with her. Noel was correct – I did need a new car. I had not driven to Canberra for eighteen years, and had no intention of doing so, but had to six times the first year, and many more since – in comfort, secure in the knowledge that my car will get me there, and that Noel and God are with me as I travel.

Catharine has been taught to travel by bus to and from her workplace. She has been lost on occasions. The first time, she got on a wrong bus and ended up in the Civic Centre. She had never been there before.

A friend asked, 'Gosh, Catharine, what did you do when you knew you were lost?'

'I cried, and I said,' – she demonstrated with her hands and eyes heavenward – '"Dad, help me, I'm lost." Then a nice man talked to me, put me on a bus and told the driver to take me back to Woden, then I walked home.'

'Well, aren't you clever?' the friend said.

'Yes, I am,' Catharine agreed. 'Mum's proud of me.'

During the Easter weekend of 1999, some family were home, Catharine among them. We attended Saturday evening Mass.

On Sunday, Catharine took me aside. 'I want Dad to be alive again!' she confided earnestly.

'I'd like that too, darling. But that can't happen,' I told her.

'Well, Jesus did!' she announced resolutely. 'Why can't Dad too?'

What could I say? 'That's because Jesus is God,' I managed, as I held her close.

She accepted my explanation and I breathed a sigh of relief.

Even though she still often comments, 'I wish Dad was alive,' she knows and accepts our loss.

On a weekend home, almost two years after his death, she said, 'We haven't been to the cemetery yet.'

I told her we could go any time she wished, concluding, 'I don't go often. I feel Dad's near me wherever I am.'

To which she responded, 'Yes, he's here in my heart, too,' placing her hand on her chest.

On one visit to the cemetery recently, she was very upset to find a small ceramic angel that she had painted and had Michael stick onto the headstone area on the first Christmas was missing.

'We'll get another one,' I promised.

Between sobs she protested, 'I painted that one for my dad.'

Whilst cleaning around Noel's grave some weeks later, I noticed an odd-shaped clod of soil with coloured pieces that was protruding from under the edge of the plants at the head of the adjoining grave. On closer inspection, I realised it was Catharine's angel, covered in dry mud. I washed it under a nearby tap and it came up as good as new. I was thrilled with my find, but had no idea how it got where it was, since I had searched for it a couple of times before. I asked the cemetery attendant if he would please glue it back in place. He did this using Liquid Nails adhesive, saying, 'It won't come off again.'

When Catharine visited for Father's Day, she was excited to see her special gift to Dad where it should be.

A few weeks later, after attending a funeral, I walked with our granddaughter, Keren, to visit her grandfather's grave. The angel was not there. As we stood in disbelief, Keren spotted a broken piece some feet away in the lawn. Looking further she retrieved six more. It had obviously been kicked by some callous person, shattering it in all directions.

As soon as we arrived home, Keren proceeded to fit and glue the angel together, hoping she had all the fragments. Only one small piece was missing from the back, so it was not noticeable. Again that special gift is back in place, with Catharine unaware of the second episode. I pray it will not be tampered with again, as it means a great deal to her.

Sending Catharine to live at L'Arche, plus the pressure to constantly bolster and encourage her to stay there, is by far the most difficult cross I have had to bear. If I was not convinced it was in her best interests, I could not keep it up. Supported by the prayers of many, and with the grace of God, we will succeed.

Catharine is spiritually strong. She has a complete faith that Dad and God are watching over her, as do I. Still I pray daily for all our children – that God keeps them safe, and that they find contentment and happiness with people they care for and who care for and understand them, as they share their lives. My consolation is in knowing that God hears our prayers, otherwise I could not let go of Catharine. There have been a few scary times over the years in trying to allow her to become independent, but she has always been safe.

The staff at each L'Arche house consists of a house coordinator and one live-in assistant, plus part-time staff, who work on a roster system, having two on duty at all times. Fran, the coordinator of the Gleden Street home, is a mature, married lady with two adult daughters. Her gentle, but firm, understanding manner brings a calming effect to the household. You must appreciate that there are very distinct needs and personalities in the four adult residents. They are also from quite different backgrounds. All the staff need to be special, caring people who are patient and kind.

Catharine, with her affectionate, extremely sensitive nature, needs constant support and affirmation, especially following so closely the loss of her father. Even though she likes and gets along with all the staff members, it is Fran on whom she relies in times of uncertainty. She often alludes to her as 'My Canberra mum.' Whenever I am concerned about Catharine's state of mind, I get much consolation by discussing my misgivings with Fran.

I have spent a few short stays at Gleden Street, and I am made very welcome by everyone, residents and staff alike. This has given me the opportunity to observe and ascertain first-hand the time, effort and expertise given to each person's particular responsibility.

One such lady is Terese, who has recently relinquished the position after seven years as the Canberra Community L'Arche Genesaret leader, an intensely demanding position. Terese is clearly drawn to people with a disability.

The assistants are often from other L'Arche communities abroad, staying different lengths of time from six months upward. The religious nuns who are carers are not addressed as 'Sister'. They have their reasons for this that I must respect. However, I cannot but regret their stand. What outstanding role models these ladies could be! I believe that, if they could observe them, more would answer their calling to religious orders.

At times, when I am feeling sorry for myself, I grieve the loss of Noel and Catharine. But, for the most part, I keep myself busy and am constantly reminded of the blessings we shared, and that he is now enjoying the rewards of a life spent knowing, loving and serving God.

The greatest legacy I have received in life is the Catholic faith of my maternal lineage, which Noel and I both shared. My fervent prayer is that our children and grandchildren come to treasure their Catholic heritage and keep their particular branch of the vine fruitful.

Catharine has ben living in Canberra for four years now. Her life is busy with work and social activities. She also does voluntary work in aged care, which she thoroughly enjoys.

On a visit with her before Christmas, Catharine and I went to Woden Plaza to complete our gift shopping. Taking charge, Catharine guided me up and down corridors and escalators, and from shop to shop, then to an eatery, where we ate lunch.

Rested and refreshed, we decided to take in a movie at the theatre complex.

'Give me your pension card, Mum. I'll shout you,' she said.

As I stood beside her at the booth, the ticket seller, a young man, asked, 'Are you her carer?'

'Yes, I suppose I am,' I answered his unexpected question.

He passed me a small form to sign, which I found discounted my entry fee.

Later, as I recalled the incident, I felt a pang of conscience for accepting the offer. Catharine had been *my* carer from the moment we had entered the door of this, for me, unfamiliar maze of shops and bustling throng. The tables had been turned. I was proud and happy to witness this growth in maturity and confidence in our girl. Again, an example of God answering our earnest prayers for her future well-being.

Even though she is not immune from the trials and tribulations that everyone encounters daily, the genuine joy and love of life Catharine radiates is infectious, and it enriches the lives of all she encounters.

How she accepts herself became clear during a recent interview on television for Down Syndrome Awareness Week 2002, when she was asked by a reporter, 'What does it mean to you to have Down syndrome? Does it make any difference to you?'

'No, it doesn't! I enjoy myself,' she answered, then added, 'Down syndrome people are special, because God makes people different. Down syndrome is a disability, and those who have it are a different kind of people.'

'So, it *is* a disability,' the reporter said.

'Yes, it *is!*' she agreed.

'You have a pretty good life,' he commented.

'Yes, I do. I enjoy myself.'

I am thankful for our immediate and extended families for the manner in which they have carried out the special mission that God has entrusted to us. We followed our instincts in the certain knowledge that each life is God-given and to be cherished.

We have been truly blessed.